RADIOGRAPHY

EXAMINATION REVIEW

RADIOGRAPHY

SEVENTH EDITION

800
Multiple-choice Questions with Explanatory Answers

William L. Leonard, MA, RT(R)
*Associate Professor of Allied Health
and
Radiography Program Director
Bergen Community College
Paramus, New Jersey*

MEDICAL EXAMINATION PUBLISHING COMPANY

Notice: The author(s) and the publisher of this volume have taken care that the information and recommendations contained herein are accurate and compatible with the standards generally accepted at the time of publication. Nevertheless, it is difficult to ensure that all the information given is entirely accurate for all circumstances. The publisher disclaims any liability, loss, or damage incurred as a consequence, directly or indirectly, of the use and application of any of the contents of this volume.

Copyright © 1991 by Appleton & Lange
Simon & Schuster Business and Professional Group

93 94 95 96 97 / 10 9 8 7 6 5 4 3 2 1

Prentice Hall International (UK) Limited, *London*
Prentice Hall of Australia Pty. Limited, *Sydney*
Prentice Hall Canada, Inc., *Toronto*
Prentice Hall Hispanoamericana, S.A., *Mexico*
Prentice Hall of India Private Limited, *New Delhi*
Prentice Hall of Japan, Inc., *Tokyo*
Simon & Schuster Asia Pte. Ltd., *Singapore*
Editora Prentice Hall do Brasil Ltda., *Rio de Janeiro*
Prentice Hall, *Englewood Cliffs, New Jersey*

ISBN 0-8385-8241-9

9 780838 582411   90000

Library of Congress Catalog Card Number: 92-083810

PRINTED IN THE UNITED STATES OF AMERICA

To my family,
Jo-Carol, Eric, Christina, and Max

Contents

Preface

Radiography graduates who have completed a comprehensive curriculum must possess a good understanding of the basic concepts in order to be effective team members in a modern radiology department. If, during their training, the students have performed the competencies required in clinical and didactic subject areas, they should have relatively minor concerns when preparing for the certification examination. Unfortunately, we all experience some degree of anxiety when we prepare for an important examination. This book is designed to assist the graduates in their final assessment and to indicate areas of strength and weakness that may require further investigation prior to the registry/licensure examination.

A profile of the five major subject areas is presented prior to each content section; cognitive skills that are measured on the actual exam evaluate levels of knowledge, comprehension, application, and analysis skills. The multiple-choice format parallels the certifying examination in design and reflects an appropriate difficulty level. The 800 questions included in this edition were developed from a review of 40 of the more standard and current textbooks adopted by radiography training programs and in compliance with topics outlined in the *American Society of Radiologic Technologists Curriculum Guide.*

This book can be used for review for the registry exam, preparation for challenge exams for college credit, and in-service programs. It also will be useful to foreign radiographers seeking certification and those individuals returning to the radiography work force who wish to do a self-evaluation. Candidates should begin preparing for the exam 10 to 12 weeks prior to the actual examination testing date. Throughout this period, and using this book as a study guide, candidates will be able to:

1. review the guidelines for test taking and apply the steps outlined
2. familiarize themselves with important formulas and theorems needed for calculations and conversions
3. examine the outlines of the major subject areas presented before each section
4. review the four cognitive levels that are tested
5. use the reference and explanatory answer sections provided for each question to promote further clarification and reinforcement

I hope that some fears and apprehensions will be alleviated and that the reader will find this book helpful in identifying areas that need additional review prior to the certification examination. I wish you success in your future endeavors in the exciting field of diagnostic radiography.

Acknowledgments

I wish to commend my lovely wife, Jo-Carol, for her patience and support in the preparation of this manuscript.

Also, I wish to express my sincere appreciation to a very special friend, Mrs. Cindy Klingner, Allied Health and Physical Education Divisional Executive Secretary, Bergen Community College, for sharing her time and computer expertise with me, in the preparation of this book.

Guidelines for Test Taking

All examinees experience some sense of anxiety when confronted with a standardized test that will assess their overall knowledge of radiography. If you have applied yourself during your training program and have command of the subjects outlined in the content specifications of your curriculum, you have little to fear. Your final task, prior to certification, is to demonstrate clearly your proficiency on a written examination. Careful preparation and test readiness are required for successful test taking. The examinee must allow sufficient time to complete an intense review, with adequate time allotted for research into unfamiliar or confusing concepts.

Once you have a thorough understanding of the knowledge required, you should apply the following steps to maximize your performance on the certification examination.

1. Prepare yourself for the certification examination by reviewing the American Registry of Radiologic Technologists (ARRT) handbook that accompanies your application for the examination. Familiarize yourself with the test format, number of questions, and scoring and weight of the questions in each section.
2. Allow yourself adequate time to study for the examination so that, instead of cramming on the night before the exam, you get a good night's sleep and feel well rested the day of the examination.
3. Allow yourself enough time to arrive at the examination site (with your admission ticket) at least 15 minutes before the examination is scheduled to commence. When planning your travel time, take into consideration traffic, bad weather, and other unexpected situations that could cause a delay. Examinees may not be admitted to the testing center once the exam session has begun.

4. You should bring the following testing materials:
   - a battery-operated calculator with which you are familiar
   - three or four #2 pencils with erasers
   - a watch to aid you in organizing your time and pacing yourself

   Books and papers of any kind may not be taken into the examination room. Scratch work may be done in the margins of the exam booklet.

5. Before beginning the examination, read all instructions carefully and scan the exam to ensure that it is complete and that the answer sheet and all pages are intact. Organize your test materials to save time and avoid errors.

6. Carefully review every word in the questions and look for key words (such as *always*, *never*, *only*, *most*, or *not*) that clarify what the question is really asking.

7. Answer the question that is asked and relate it to your knowledge of the content. After reading the problem statement, anticipate the answer before you begin reading the options. Try to put the question and the answer in your own words to test your comprehension.

8. Read each distracter carefully and try to compare options for similarities and differences.

9. Eliminate poor or absurd distracters to increase your probability of selecting the correct answer. If you are not absolutely sure of an answer, make an educated guess. It is to your advantage to answer every question.

10. Relate each possible or feasible option to the stem question.

11. If you should draw a blank, relax and simply place a check in the exam booklet. Do not waste time on an extremely difficult or unfamiliar question. The more anxious you become, the more it will affect your overall test performance. Move on and come back to the question later. The rest of the test may provide you with information that may help when you reread the problem question a second time. Watch your answer key for transposition errors.

12. First impressions are usually correct; a large part of subconscious knowledge does come into awareness during an exam. Do not change your answers unless you misread the question, missed a relevant fact, or, after review, discovered that you inadvertently darkened the wrong box on the answer key. Completely erase the wrong answer when changing the key.

13. Know how the examination is scored. If a question is not answered, it will be marked wrong. If two answers are recorded by the sensor, the question will be marked wrong. It is better to guess at an answer than to leave a blank.

14. Use the full three hours to complete your examination. Use any extra time to review your answers, especially those you checked and problems involving calculations, decimal points, and formulas.
15. Set realistic expectations. Do not expect to get all questions correct.
16. After the exam, assess your overall performance. Remember, even though you may be test-taking wise, you must have command of the subject matter.

Cognitive Levels

Specific cognitive abilities are required as practitioners make judgments in actual clinical situations. The ARRT examination evaluates these critical intellectual processes, including knowledge, comprehension, application, and analysis.

Knowledge

The knowledge level emphasizes the process of remembering. The examinee recalls facts about principles, concepts, theories, terms, or procedures. In answering a knowledge question the examinee does little more than recognize the appropriate response from among those offered. The knowledge cognitive level represents the most basic kind of mastery over subject matter and requires you to define, identify, or select.

The following is an example of a knowledge question:

1. Which of the following is **NOT** a part of the cranium?
   A. Dorsum sellae
   B. Hyoid
   C. Perpendicular plate
   D. Anterior clinoid process
   Answer: B.

Comprehension

The comprehension level presupposes recall ability and further requires understanding or interpretation of the subject matter. The question must present some kind of communication that is to be comprehended or translated. These questions require interpretation, explanation, differentiation, or prediction; they test your intellectual ability to comprehend information.

The following is an example of a comprehension question:

2. A lateral skull is normally exposed at 300 mA, 1/5 second, 75 kVp, 40-in SID. What new mAs would be needed to maintain density if the kVp were reduced to 65 kVp?
   A. 30 mAs
   B. 60 mAs
   C. 120 mAs
   D. 240 mAs
   Answer: C.

Application

The application level requires that the examinee rearrange material that has been learned in order to select the answer. This involves the application of laws, rules, methods, principles, concepts, and theories. This comprehension information is adapted to new and real situations.

The following is an example of a application question:

1. Which of the following radiographic techniques would produce the highest incidence of direct exposure to the fetus?
   A. 300 mA, 1/2 second, 65 kVp, 36-in SID
   B. 400 mA, 1/15 second, 80 kVp, 42-in SID
   C. 500 mA, 1/30 second, 85 kVp, 44-in SID
   D. 600 mA, 1/60 second, 95 kVp, 46-in SID
   Answer: A.

Analysis

The analysis level assumes abilities in all three previous cognitive skills. The examinee must be able to break down material into its component parts in order to understand its basic structure. Test items that evaluate at the analysis level require the ability to analyze, evaluate, differentiate, or interpret data from a variety of sources.

An example of an analysis question is as follows.

1. An abdomen radiograph produces 240 mR at a 20-in SID. How many milliroentgens would be produced at a 40-in SID after passage through an additional 2 HVL?
   A. 15 mR
   B. 30 mR
   C. 60 mR
   D. 120 mR
   Answer: A.

Important Formulas

A function is a unit of density that will double the density (+1) or cut the density in half (-1). Functions relate to:

1. Milliamperage (2 × or ½ mAs) ⎱
2. Exposure time (2 × or ½ mAs) ⎰
3. Kilovoltage (15%; 15% kV = 50% mAs)
4. Screen speed (slow, medium, high, rare-earth)
5. 5 cm of patient thickness (60 to 80 kV range)

mAs distance relationship: $\dfrac{mAs_1}{mAs_2} = \dfrac{D_1^2}{D_2^2}$

R = H/D (R = grid ratio; H = height of lead strips; D = width of the space between the strips)

Grid conversion factors (in mAs):
5:1 = 2 × mAs   10:1 = 5 × mAs
6:1 = 3 × mAs   12:1 = 5 × mAs
8:1 = 4 × mAs   16:1 = 6 × mAs

New mAs = Original mAs × $\dfrac{\text{New grid conversion factor}}{\text{Original grid conversion factor}}$

Degree of magnification = $\dfrac{\text{Image width}}{\text{Object width}}$

Magnification factor = $\dfrac{\text{SID}}{\text{SOD}}$

Image unsharpness = FSS × $\dfrac{\text{OID}}{\text{SOD}}$

Heat units (HU) = mA × time × kVp
3 phase, 6 pulse = ×1.35
3 phase, 12 pulse = ×1.41
Maximum permissible dose:
MPD = 5 (N–18) rem or 50 (N–18) mSv

Whole Body	Quarterly	Weekly
5 rem/yr	1.25 rem/3 mo	0.01 rem/wk
5,000 mrem/yr	1200 mrem/3 mo	100 mrem/wk
50 mSv/yr	12.5 mSv/3 mo	

Skin	Hands	Forearms
15 rem/yr	75 rem/yr	30 rem/yr
15,000 mrem/yr	75,000 mrem/yr	30,000 mrem/yr
150 mSv/yr	750 mSv/yr	300 mSv/yr

Fetus in utero = 0.5 rem or 5 mSv (during entire gestation)
1 gray (Gy) = 100 rad or 1 rad = 0.01 Gy
1 seivert (Sv) = 100 rem or 1,000 mSv

1 Radiation Protection

The major subject areas covered in radiation protection include the following.

1. Radiation protection of the patient and radiographer with emphasis on women of childbearing age, male patients, pediatric patients, and the pregnant radiographer.

2. Maximum permissible dosages (MPDs) for various population groups, units of measure, dose effects, long-term effects, somatic and genetic dose indicators, special concerns, and calculations involving the MPD formula.

3. Minimizing patient exposure, including adjustment of technical factors, shielding, beam restriction, filtration, grids, patient positioning, film and screen combinations, phototiming, air gap procedures, and special protective devices and measures.

4. The effects of ionizing radiation on various body structures, radiosensitive organs, and high-risk examinations.

5. Radiation protection of the radiographer, including scatter, leakage, and primary beam exposure. Various methods of protection involving routine diagnostic procedures, portable examinations, and fluoroscopic and special procedure studies.

6. Federal agencies and regulations that relate to the controlling of ionizing radiation to include room design and barriers. Recommendations from NCRP regarding protection by use of lead aprons, gloves, and other protective devices.

7. Radiation monitors, detection and various radiation interactions with matter, basic properties of radiation, units of measure, and federal recommendations.

8. Radiation biology, background sources of radiation, and radiation effects on certain tissues, especially reproductive organs and their response level to irradiation.

DIRECTIONS (Questions 1–150): Each of the questions or incomplete statements below is followed by four suggested answers or completions. Select the **one** that is best in each case.

1. Which of the following radiographic techniques would exhibit the **LEAST** amount of radiation exposure to the pregnant patient?
   A. 200 mA, 1/2 sec, 65 kVp, par-speed screens
   B. 400 mA, 1/10 sec, 80 kVp, high-speed screens
   C. 100 mA, 3/4 sec, 60 kVp, par-speed screens
   D. 75 mA, 4/5 sec, 65 kVp, par-speed screens

2. Which of the following radiographic techniques would be most harmful to the fetus in a single radiographic exposure to the mother's abdomen?
   A. 200 mA, 1/2 sec, 65 kVp, par-speed screens
   B. 400 mA, 0.10 sec, 85 kVp, high-speed screens
   C. 600 mA, 0.40 sec, 70 kVp, medium-speed screens
   D. 100 mA, 1/20 sec, 90 kVp, high-speed screens

3. Which of the following will help reduce exposure to the patient?
   1. High kV, low mAs
   2. Collimation
   3. Filtration
   A. 1 and 2 only
   B. 1 and 3 only
   C. 2 and 3 only
   D. 1, 2, and 3

4. Which of the following will provide radiation protection for the patient and also preserve radiographic contrast?
   1. Close collimation
   2. Change par- to high-speed screen and decrease mAs
   3. High kV, low mAs techniques
   A. 1 and 2 only
   B. 1 and 3 only
   C. 2 and 3 only
   D. 1, 2, and 3

5. What is the MPD for a pregnant woman?
   A. 0.25 rem
   B. 0.5 rem
   C. 1.5 rem
   D. 2.5 rem

6. The ten-day rule states that all nonemergency x-ray examinations on women of reproductive capacity should be
   A. scheduled at ten-day intervals
   B. scheduled ten days before their next menstruation
   C. delayed until ten days after menstruation
   D. scheduled during the ten-day period following the onset of menstruation

7. With patient safety as the **MOST** important factor, select the screen that would best satisfy this requirement.
   A. Detail
   B. Medium speed
   C. Hi plus
   D. Rare earth

8. The **DECREASE** in exposure rate of radiation caused by passage through material is known as
   A. absorbed dose
   B. attenuation
   C. remnant radiation
   D. depth dosage

9. Which of the following is **NOT** considered part of inherent filtration?
   A. The glass envelope of the tube
   B. Housing materials
   C. The oil insulation
   D. Aluminum

10. A 1-mm lead apron worn by a pregnant technologisst will attenuate a 75-kVp beam approximately
    A. 30% to 40%
    B. 50% to 60%
    C. 80% to 90%
    D. 98% to 99%

11. When a beam of 80 mAs passes through 3 HVL the new intensity would be
    A. 10 mAs
    B. 20 mAs
    C. 40 mAs
    D. 60 mAs

12. The primary purpose of a filter is to
    A. eliminate long-wavelength photons
    B. restrict secondary radiation
    C. preserve contrast
    D. enhance definition

13. The half-value layer may be defined as that amount of filtration which will reduce the original intensity by
    A. 25%
    B. 50%
    C. 75%
    D. 100%

14. The inherent filtration in aluminum of a general-purpose x-ray tube is usually about
    A. 0.5 mm
    B. 1.25 mm
    C. 1.5 mm
    D. 2.5 mm

15. Which of the following is an example of a compensating filter?
    A. Potter-Bucky diaphragm
    B. Penetrometer
    C. Inherent filter
    D. Graduated aluminum wedge

16. An occupational worker may receive an exposure of 25 rems to the hands and feet during a
    A. one-week period
    B. three-week period
    C. 13-week period
    D. one-year period

17. Radiographers who begin training prior to age 18 are limited to a yearly MPD of
    A. 100 mR (1 mSv)
    B. 500 mR (5 mSv)
    C. 1,000 mR (10 mSv)
    D. 3,000 mR (30 mSv)

18. The MPD for one year to the lungs is
    A. 5 rems
    B. 15 rems
    C. 30 rems
    D. 75 rems

19. Which of the following radiographic techniques would deliver the lowest patient dosage?
    A. 300 mA, 1/6 sec, 70 kV, 1.0 mm, Al filter
    B. 150 mA, 1/3 sec, 75 kV, 1.5 mm, Al filter
    C. 100 mA, 1/2 sec, 82 kV, 2.0 mm, Al filter
    D. 100 mA, 1/4 sec, 90 kV, 3.0 mm, Al filter

20. In which of the following body areas is the MPD 5 rems for a 13-week period?
    1. Forearms
    2. Lungs
    3. Thyroid
    A. 1 only
    B. 1 and 2 only
    C. 2 and 3 only
    D. 1, 2, and 3

21. The radiation dose necessary to cause skin erythema in 50% of exposed persons is about
    A. 50 rads (0.5 Gy)
    B. 600 rads (6 Gy)
    C. 8,000 rads (80 Gy)
    D. 10,000 rads (100 Gy)

22. The roentgen is defined by the
    A. degree of blackening of a film
    B. amount of fluorescence of a crystal
    C. number of ions produced in air
    D. number of ions produced in any medium

23. Which of the changes in the following technique would result in highest patient exposure? 300 mA, 1/5 sec, 80 kV, 40 in FFD, 5:1 grid
    A. Change from 80 kV to 90 kV
    B. Change to 48 in FFD
    C. Use 30 mAs at 92 kV
    D. Convert from 6:1 grid to 16:1 grid

24. If the intensity of a particular x-ray beam is 450 mR at 40 in, what would its intensity be at 10 feet?
    A. 25 mR
    B. 50 mR
    C. 125 mR
    D. 225 mR

25. Which of the following units of measure are used to express absorbed dose?
       1. Rad
       2. Gray
       3. Roentgen
    A. 1 and 2 only
    B. 1 and 3 only
    C. 2 and 3 only
    D. 1, 2, and 3

26. 5 rem equal
   A. 5 mSv
   B. 50 mSv
   C. 500 mSv
   D. 5,000 mSv

27. The unit of dose equivalent that is used to express radiation exposure to living tissue is the
   A. roentgen
   B. rad
   C. rem
   D. erg

28. The MPD for radiation workers' whole body exposure is
   1. 5 rem/yr
   2. 1.2 rem in a single 13-week period
   3. 0.1 rem/wk
   A. 1 and 2 only
   B. 1 and 3 only
   C. 2 and 3 only
   D. 1, 2, and 3

29. If a radiation worker were to receive an exposure of 3 rem during the first three months of a calendar year, what would be the maximum additional exposure he could receive during the remainder of that year?
   A. No exposure
   B. 2 rem
   C. 3 rem
   D. 5 rem

30. If a radiation intensity is measured at 512 mR at a distance of 4 in, what would be the intensity at 32 in?
   A. 8 mR
   B. 84 mR
   C. 360 mR
   D. 612 mR

31. If the intensity of radiation from an x-ray tube is 20 R/min at a distance of 72 in, what would the intensity be at a distance of 48 in?
    A. 15 R/min
    B. 25 R/min
    C. 45 R/min
    D. 80 R/min

32. The output intensity of a fluoroscopic tube is 600 mR/h at 0.5 m from the tube. If the radiographer stands at 1.0 m from the tube during 20 minutes of fluoroscopy, what is the total occupational exposure?
    A. 25 mR
    B. 50 mR
    C. 150 mR
    D. 300 mR

33. The difference in tissue absorption can be scaled to radiographic requirements by proper selection of
    A. mAs
    B. kV
    C. focal spot size
    D. distance

34. If a chest radiograph produced 120 mR at 72 in, how many mR would be produced at 18 in?
    A. 240 mR
    B. 480 mR
    C. 960 mR
    D. 1,920 mR

35. How many amperes are equal to 100 mA?
    A. 0.001
    B. 0.01
    C. 0.1
    D. 1.0

36. A radiographer receives 150 mR during 2 minutes of fluoroscopy while standing 6 feet from the unit. What is the approximate exposure the radiographer would receive if she/he stands 2 feet from the unit for 30 seconds?
    A. 1,350 mR
    B. 340 mR
    C. 1,000 mR
    D. 500 mR

37. The difference between the roentgen (R) and the rad is that the rad represents the unit of
    A. exposure
    B. absorbed dosage
    C. filtration
    D. wavelength

38. The MPD for the eyes is the same as for the
    1. skin
    2. whole body
    3. gonads
    A. 1 and 2 only
    B. 1 and 3 only
    C. 2 and 3 only
    D. 1, 2, and 3

39. The common measuring unit to express exposure to radiation interactions with air is the
    A. erg
    B. joule
    C. roentgen
    D. sievert

40. One rad equals 100 ergs of energy absorbed in 1 g of
    A. soft tissue
    B. bone
    C. muscle
    D. any absorber

41. The MPD in millirems per year for whole-body radiation for an occupational worker is
   A. 0.5
   B. 50.0
   C. 500
   D. 5,000

42. Which of the following effects would **NOT** occur in the 200 to 1,000 rad exposure level?
   A. Gonadal atrophy
   B. Bone marrow hypoplasia
   C. Lymphoid atrophy
   D. Brain necrosis

43. Central nervous system (CNS) death requires radiation dosages in rads of
   A. 50
   B. 500
   C. 5,000
   D. 50,000

44. The unit of absorbed dose, the rad, is determined by which one of the following?
   A. Biologic effect of the radiation
   B. Counts recorded per minute
   C. Energy deposited in a volume of matter
   D. Number of ions produced in a given volume of air

45. A 35-year-old radiographer who has accumulated 10 R will **NOT** exceed his/her MPD until receiving
   A. 75 R
   B. 125 mR
   C. 750 mR
   D. 1,050 mR

46. The whole-body MPD does **NOT** apply to the
    A. head
    B. lens of the eye
    C. gonads
    D. skin

47. The dose rate at 50 cm from a source is 75 mR/h. What is the dose rate in mR/h at 90 cm?
    A. 23.1
    B. 24.3
    C. 26.7
    D. 28.8

48. Which one of the following determines the radiation quality of any given x-ray beam?
    A. Heat of the filament
    B. kVp
    C. mAs
    D. Size of focal spot

49. The MPD for human skin per year is
    A. 5,000 mrem/yr
    B. 15,000 mrem/yr
    C. 30,000 mrem/yr
    D. 25,000 mrem/yr

50. During a radiographer's pregnancy, her exposure should **NOT** exceed
    A. 300 mrem
    B. 500 mrem
    C. 1,000 mrem
    D. 5,000 mrem

51. The MPD for a male occupationally exposed worker is
    A. 0.05 rem/yr
    B. 0.5 rem/yr
    C. 5.0 rem/yr
    D. 50.0 rem/yr

52. If a technologist begins to practice radiation protection by standing in the fluoroscopic room half as much as he previously did, and increases his standing from 3 to 6 feet when he is in the room, how much will this technologist **DECREASE** his radiation dose?
A. 1/2
B. 1/4
C. 1/8
D. 1/12

53. During fluoroscopic examinations in which the patient is lying on the x-ray table, the radiographer should normally stand
A. behind the radiologist
B. to the radiologist's side
C. in the control booth
D. on the opposite side of the table from the radiologist

54. If 4,000 photons are measured at a distance of 1 m, how many photons will be measured at a distance of 2 m after they have passed through an absorber whose thickness is equal to 2 HVL?
A. 250
B. 500
C. 1,000
D. 2,000

55. Which of the following protective devices must have a minimum of 0.15 mm of lead equivalent?
A. Filters
B. Primary barriers
C. Fluoroscopic screen curtain
D. Tube housing

56. If exposure factors of 200 mA, 1/10 sec, 80 kV at a 72-in FFD produce 40 mR, what mR would be produced at 400 mA, 1/20 sec, 80 kV, at 36 in?
A. 40 mR
B. 120 mR
C. 160 mR
D. 240 mR

57. When lead aprons are employed during fluoroscopy, film badges should be worn
   A. outside the apron level of the waist
   B. inside the apron level of the waist
   C. inside the apron level of the neck
   D. outside the apron level of the neck

58. The effect of radiation exposure that appears during an individual's lifetime is called
   A. genetic
   B. somatic
   C. carcinogenic
   D. occupational

59. On the basis of radiation protection guides, which of the following is permitted the smallest accumulated radiation dose?
   A. Lungs
   B. Thyroid gland
   C. Eye lens
   D. Hands, forearms, and feet

60. Which of the following x-ray beams possesses the highest quality?
   A. 70 kV with 2.0 mm AL filter
   B. 90 kV with 3.0 mm AL filter
   C. 80 kV with 1.5 mm AL filter
   D. 85 kV with 2.5 mm AL filter

61. If a radiographer received a dosage of 10 mR/h at a distance of 100 cm, exposure can be reduced to 2.5 mR/h at which of the following distances?
   A. 200 cm
   B. 400 cm
   C. 600 cm
   D. 800 cm

62. Which of the following types of cells is **MOST** radioresistant?
    A. Lymphocytes
    B. Spermatogonia
    C. Erythroblasts
    D. Endothelial

63. One gray equals
    A. 1/100 of a rad
    B. 1/10 of a rad
    C. 10 rads
    D. 100 rads

64. Which of the following radiographic techniques would provide the **LEAST** amount of exposure to the patient?
    A. 30 mAs at 120 kV
    B. 100 mAs at 85 kV
    C. 50 mAs at 65 kV
    D. 200 mAs at 75 kV

65. A measurement of 0.2 R is equal to
    A. 0.002 mR
    B. 20 mR
    C. 200 mR
    D. 2,000 mR

66. Which of the following cell types falls into the high radiosensitive category?
    1. Spermatids
    2. Erythroblasts
    3. Lymphocytes
    A. 1 only
    B. 1 and 2 only
    C. 2 and 3 only
    D. 1, 2, and 3

67. What percentage of molecular composition does the human body contain in protein?
    A. 1%
    B. 2%
    C. 15%
    D. 40%

68. What syndrome normally appears following a whole-body exposure of 1,000 to 5,000 rads?
    A. Gastrointestinal
    B. Hematological
    C. Prodromal
    D. Epilation

69. The genetic effects of radiation occur in an irradiated
    A. ovum
    B. embryo
    C. fetus
    D. neonate

70. The last and most severe stage in the acute radiation syndrome (radiation sickness) involves
    A. neurological symptoms
    B. erythema
    C. cytogenic damage
    D. nausea and diarrhea

71. Which one of the following would be a long-term effect of exposure to ionizing radiation?
    A. Carcinogenesis
    B. Diarrhea
    C. Fever
    D. Nausea

72. Which of the following is a somatic effect of radiation?
   1. Leukemia
   2. Nausea
   3. Cataracts
   A. 1 and 2 only
   B. 1 and 3 only
   C. 2 and 3 only
   D. 1, 2, and 3

73. Which of the following exams would result in the highest bone marrow dose for a 10-year-old child?
   A. Extremity
   B. Skull
   C. Pelvis
   D. Abdomen

74. Which of the following tissues is **MOST** radioresistant?
   A. Nervous tissue
   B. Blood-forming tissue
   C. Intestinal crypt cells
   D. Mucosal linings of organs

75. Which of the following examinations would have the highest estimated gonad dose for the pregnant patient?
   A. Lumbar spine
   B. IVP
   C. Pelvis
   D. Upper GI

76. Which of the following dosages to the total body would cause the gastrointestinal syndrome in 4 to 10 days?
   A. 100 rads
   B. 200 to 500 rads
   C. 600 to 800 rads
   D. 1,000 to 5,000 rads

77. Which of the following cell types has a low radiosensitivity?
    A. Spermatogonia
    B. Chondrocytes
    C. Fibroblasts
    D. Lymphocytes

78. Which nucleic acid is important in human metabolism?
    1. Carbonucleic
    2. Deoxyribonucleic
    3. Ribonucleic
    A. 1 only
    B. 1 and 2 only
    C. 2 and 3 only
    D. 1, 2, and 3

79. Which of the following radiations would be the **LEAST** penetrating?
    A. Alpha
    B. Beta
    C. Gamma
    D. X-rays

80. If it is necessary for a patient to be held by another person during radiography, the best choice of person (assuming all persons considered are competent) would be
    A. an older adult relative
    B. a young adult relative
    C. a radiologic technologist
    D. a radiologist

81. During a four-minute fluoroscopic examination, the survey meter shows that the technologist is exposed to 240 mR/h. What is the exposure in mR during this procedure?
    A. 16
    B. 48
    C. 60
    D. 80

82. The hematologic syndrome occurs from radiation dosages in the range of
   A. 0 to 100 rads
   B. 200 to 1,000 rads
   C. 1,000 to 5,000 rads
   D. 5,000 to 10,000 rads

83. Which of the following cell types is high in radiosensitivity?
   A. Lymphocytes
   B. Endothelial cells
   C. Chondrocytes
   D. Fibroblasts

84. Which of the following examinations would have the highest exposure risk for a female patient?
   A. Lumbar spine
   B. Abdomen
   C. Pelvis
   D. Skull

85. If a pregnant radiographer had her choice of where to be assigned within the radiology department, the safest place would be in
   A. special procedures
   B. IVP
   C. GI
   D. Portables

86. The "bone marrow syndrome" is also known as the
   A. hemagioma syndrome
   B. hemarthosis syndrome
   C. hematohidrosis syndrome
   D. hematopoietic syndrome

87. What is the exposure rate delivered when 60 mAs produces 300 mR?
   A. 3 mR/mAs
   B. 5 mR/mAs
   C. 10 mR/mAs
   D. 20 mR/mAs

88. Which of the following is **MOST** sensitive to the somatic effects of radiation exposure?
   A. The fetus
   B. A small child
   C. A mature adult of reproductive age
   D. An elderly individual

89. Which of the following is considered a late or delayed radiation effect on humans?
   A. Cytogenetic damage
   B. Leukemia
   C. Local tissue damage
   D. Hematologic depression

90. Which of the following body tissues is the **MOST** radiosensitive?
   A. Central nervous system
   B. Blood forming organs
   C. Solid visceral organs
   D. Muscular organs

91. How much equivalent aluminum filtration does the glass window in most x-ray tubes provide?
   A. 0.25 mm Al
   B. 0.5 mm Al
   C. 1.0 mm Al
   D. 1.5 mm Al

92. Which of the following statements regarding the laws of radiosensitivity should be considered **CORRECT**?
   1. The younger the tissue, the more radiosensitive it is
   2. Mature cells are the most radioresistant
   3. When metabolic activity is high, so is radiosensitivity
   A. 1 only
   B. 1 and 2 only
   C. 2 and 3 only
   D. 1, 2, and 3

93. Which of the following cell types is high in radiosensitivity?
   A. Chondrocytes
   B. Erythroblasts
   C. Spermatids
   D. Osteoblasts

94. Humans are most sensitive to radiation
   A. immediately after birth
   B. in the early developmental years
   C. before birth
   D. in old age

95. A major disadvantage of soft tissue radiography is
   A. long scale contrast
   B. wide penumbra
   C. high patient dosage
   D. object magnification

96. The x-ray attenuation at 75 kVp for a protective apron with 0.5 mm lead equivalence is
   A. 55%
   B. 66%
   C. 88%
   D. 99%

97. Lipid molecules are composed of
   1. glycerol
   2. fatty acids
   3. enzymes
   A. 1 only
   B. 1 and 2 only
   C. 2 and 3 only
   D. 1, 2, and 3

98. Epilation refers to
   A. the growth rate of a tumor
   B. malignant growth
   C. loss of hair
   D. metabolic imbalance

99. Which of the following is **TRUE** concerning oxygen tension and how it relates to tissue sensitivity?
   A. The higher the oxygen tension, the greater the sensitivity
   B. The lower the oxygen tension, the greater the sensitivity
   C. The higher the oxygen tension, the lower the sensitivity
   D. Oxygen tension and tissue sensitivity depend upon body temperature

100. The required shielding for the average radiographic tube housing is
   A. 0.5 mm tungsten
   B. 1 mm rhenium-steel
   C. 1.5 mm lead
   D. 2.5 mm aluminum

101. Which of the following radiographic units would be **MOST** efficient in minimizing patient exposure?
   A. Three phase, rectified six pulse
   B. Single phase, unrectified
   C. Three phase, unrectified
   D. Three phase, rectified 12 pulse

102. High-speed intensifying screens contain crystals that are
   A. large
   B. small
   C. medium
   D. inert

103. The use of high-speed intensifying screens will
   A. reduce radiographic exposure time
   B. reduce scatter radiation
   C. decrease contrast
   D. increase definition

104. The halide present in the film emulsion is silver
   A. nitrate
   B. sulfite
   C. acetate
   D. bromide

105. What is the estimated average exposure per film at skin entrance for a kidneys, ureter, bladder (KUB) film?
A. 120 mR
B. 670 mR
C. 980 mR
D. 1,320 mR

106. What percentage of body tissue is bone marrow?
A. 2.9
B. 4.2
C. 5.8
D. 7.7

107. What type of screen will yield the **BEST** resolution?
A. Ultra-detail
B. Par
C. High plus
D. Rare earth

108. Which of the following is **NOT** a rare-earth phosphor?
A. Gadolinium
B. Zinc sulfide
C. Lanthanum
D. Terbium

109. What is the color emitted by rare-earth screens made of lanthanum and gadolinium?
A. Violet
B. Blue
C. Green
D. Ultraviolet

110. Fast films and intensifying screens enable the use of a
A. higher kV range
B. shorter OFD
C. lower mAs
D. longer SID

111. The thickness of an x-ray film base is approximately
   A. 0.2 mm
   B. 0.5 mm
   C. 1.0 mm
   D. 2.0 mm

112. How much more exposure is required when using nonscreen film in a cardboard holder than screen film in a screen cassette?
   A. Two times
   B. 3 to 5 times
   C. 8 to 10 times
   D. 20 to 30 times

113. Lithium fluoride crystals are found in a
   A. film badge
   B. pocket ionization chamber
   C. thermoluminescent dosimeter (TLD)
   D. cutie pie

114. After the primary beam emerges from the patient, it is called
   A. scattered radiation
   B. secondary radiation
   C. incident radiation
   D. remnant radiation

115. The term TLD refers to a
   A. measure of radiation intensity
   B. type of personnel monitor
   C. biological radiation response
   D. equipment calibration instrument

116. Which of the following are units of measure used to express the absorbed dose in man?
    1. Rem
    2. Rad
    3. Sievert
    A. 1 and 2 only
    B. 1 and 3 only
    C. 2 and 3 only
    D. 1, 2, and 3

117. Which of the following are advantages to using the TLD rather than the film badge?
    1. Wide exposure range detectable
    2. Direct reading available at any time
    3. Response similar to that of human tissue
    A. 1 only
    B. 1 and 2 only
    C. 2 and 3 only
    D. 1, 2, and 3

118. When a photon reacts with an electron, and the resulting photon has the same energy level but moves in a different direction, it is referred to as
    A. photoelectric absorption
    B. unmodified scattering
    C. Compton effect
    D. annihilation reaction

119. Photoelectric effect ALWAYS results in
    A. total absorption of the incident photon
    B. release of a recoil electron
    C. creation of an electron and a positron
    D. formation of a proton and a neutron

120. In the diagnostic energy range, absorption of radiation using diagnostic machines is known as
    A. Compton absorption
    B. photoelectric absorption
    C. annihilation effect
    D. pair production

121. What are x-rays called that have undergone a change in direction after interactions with atoms?
    A. Scattered
    B. Primary
    C. Secondary
    D. Remnant

122. What type of interaction between matter and radiation does **NOT** occur in the normal diagnostic energy range?
    A. Photoelectric effect
    B. Compton effect
    C. Pair production
    D. Unmodified scattering

123. Which interaction delivers the highest exposure to the radiographer during a radiographic procedure?
    A. Classical scattering
    B. Compton effect
    C. Pair production
    D. Photoelectric effect

124. Unmodified scatter takes place when
    A. an x-ray photon ejects an electron
    B. a 1.02-meV x-ray photon enters an electric field
    C. all the energy is transferred to the electron
    D. a low-energy x-ray photon collides with an atom and rebounds

125. The Compton effect is characterized by
    A. no transfer of energy on collision
    B. part transfer of energy on collision
    C. total absorption of energy on collision
    D. the absence of secondary radiation

126. Which of the following monitors is considered the **MOST** accurate?
   A. Film badge
   B. TLD
   C. Photoemission
   D. Ion counter

127. During Compton interaction, the incident x-ray energy is
   1. partially absorbed
   2. shared by the photon and Compton electron
   3. absorbed more in higher atomic number materials
   A. 1 only
   B. 2 only
   C. 1 and 2 only
   D. 1, 2, and 3

128. The metal filters contained in the film badge are generally composed of
   A. aluminum or lead
   B. aluminum or copper
   C. zinc or copper
   D. lithium fluoride

129. The phenomenon on which **MOST** radiation measuring instruments depends is
   A. ionization
   B. luminescence
   C. bremsstrahlung
   D. thermionic emission

130. What lead equivalent in an apron should a pregnant technologist wear?
   A. 0.25 mm
   B. 0.5 mm
   C. 1.0 mm
   D. 1.5 mm

131. What is the name of the radiation that is emitted by atoms after having absorbed x-rays?
    A. Primary
    B. Secondary
    C. Scattered
    D. Remnant

132. Gonadal exposure should be minimized in order to prevent
    A. somatic effects
    B. genetic damage
    C. erythema
    D. cataracts

133. Which of the following is an **INCORRECT** breakdown of body composition according to tissue constituents?
    A. Muscle (43%)
    B. Fat (14%)
    C. Blood (12.4%)
    D. Skeleton (10%)

134. The final segment of mitosis is called
    A. telophase
    B. prophase
    C. interphase
    D. anaphase

135. Which of the following cell types has a high radiosensitivity?
    A. Spermatogonia
    B. Chondrocytes
    C. Osteoblasts
    D. Fibroblasts

136. Which of the following is **NOT** a clinical sign and symptom of the gastrointestinal syndrome?
    A. Lethargy
    B. Vasculitis
    C. Leukopenia
    D. Anemia

137. During the prodromal stage of radiation exposure, the patient will experience
  A. anemia
  B. nausea
  C. edema
  D. ataxia

138. Approximately 15% of the molecular composition of the body is
  A. lipids
  B. protein
  C. nucleic acids
  D. carbohydrates

139. Which statement is **INCORRECT** regarding radiosensitivity and cell type?
  A. Spermatogonia cells are highly radiosensitive
  B. Nerve cells have low radiosensitivity
  C. Muscle cells have low radiosensitivity
  D. Chondrocytes have intermediate radiosensitivity

140. Which of the following does **NOT** secrete hormones?
  A. Pancreas
  B. Pituitary
  C. Liver
  D. Gonads

141. The atomic composition of the body shows that 60% is made up of
  A. nitrogen
  B. hydrogen
  C. oxygen
  D. carbon

142. The genetic female cells are called the
  A. oogonium
  B. codon
  C. spermatogonium
  D. ribosome

143. Which of the following contains all the hereditary information representing a cell?
   A. Ribonucleic acid (RNA)
   B. Deoxyribonucleic acid (DNA)
   C. Nucleotide
   D. Pyrimidines

144. Which of the following is **MOST** radiosensitive?
   A. Granulocytes
   B. Basal cells
   C. Reticulocytes
   D. Erythroblasts

145. The supporting and binding tissue around an active cell is called the
   A. stroma
   B. endothelium
   C. outer layer
   D. periphery

146. Leakage radiation from the x-ray tube should **NOT** be more than
   A. 10 mR/h at 1/2 m
   B. 100 mR/h at 1 m
   C. 100 mR/h at 3 m
   D. 1000 mR/h at 1 m

147. The film badge **CANNOT** monitor the presence of
   A. gamma rays
   B. x-rays
   C. alpha rays
   D. low energy beta rays

148. When dealing with kilovoltage in excess of 250 kV, which of the following materials usually is used as a protective barrier?
   A. Brick
   B. Lead
   C. Plaster
   D. Concrete

149. What is the MPD to the eye lens in a 13-week period?
   A. 1.25 rems
   B. 5.0 rems
   C. 7.5 rems
   D. 10.0 rems

150. What body parts can tolerate in 13 weeks 25 rems, according to the MPD?
   1. Forearm
   2. Hands
   3. Feet
   A. 1 only
   B. 1 and 2 only
   C. 2 and 3 only
   D. 1, 2, and 3

Explanatory Answers

1. B.   A technique of lowest mAs and highest kV would be the least harmful to the fetus. (Ref. 31, p. 141)

2. C.   Fetal damage is greatest at high mAs, low kVp techniques. Low mAs, high kV, and high filtration produce lower patient dosage. (Ref. 31, p. 141)

3. D.   To control radiation exposure, three of the basic radiation control principles are to utilize high kV, low mAs techniques, collimate to the smallest field size, and utilize filters. (Ref. 6, p. 10)

4. A.   Good contrast is demonstrated with close collimation and usage of a higher-speed screen. This will also reduce patient dosage. (Ref. 6, p. 10)

5. B.   Under occupational radiation dose-limits, the MPD for the fetus in utero should not exceed 0.5 rem during the entire period of gestation. (Ref. 31, p. 56)

6. D.   The ICRP has suggested a "ten-day rule," since it is improbable that a woman would be pregnant during the first ten days following the onset of menstruation. This rule suggests that abdominal x-rays be postponed unless immediate illness is present. (Ref. 31, p. 58)

7. D.   When rare-earth screens are used, the mAs can be reduced by approximately 50%. (Ref. 6, p. 251)

8. B.   The total reduction in the number of x-rays remaining in an x-ray beam following penetration through a given thickness of matter is called attenuation. (Ref. 6, p. 170)

9. D.   Aluminum is used as the added filter and usually is 2 to 3 mm thick. (Ref. 6, p. 179)

10. D.   The x-ray attenuations for a 1.0 mm Pb apron are: 99.9% at 50 kVp, 99% at 75 kVp, and 94% at 100 kVp. (Ref. 6, p. 589)

11. A. 3 HVL = 1/8 of the original beam: 80 mAs to 40 mAs; 40 mAs to 20 mAs; 20 mAs to 10 mAs. (Ref. 6, p. 177)

12. A. Quality is changed by filtration, and exposure rate is always decreased by filtration because some long-wave, low-energy photons are attenuated. (Ref. 29, p. 208)

13. B. The HVL of an x-ray beam is defined as the thickness of a specific material which reduces the exposure rate to half, or 50%, of its initial value. (Ref. 29, p. 179)

14. A. This 0.5 mm of Al equivalent is made up by the glass envelope of the x-ray tube. (Ref. 6, p. 178)

15. D. The graduated aluminum wedge, or barium plastic compound filter, is used in radiographing parts of the body that differ greatly in thickness or density, so as to record them with more uniform density on a single film. (Ref. 29, p. 423)

16. C. According to standards introduced by the ICRU, 25 rem is the MPD for the hands and feet in a 13-week period. (Ref. 29, p. 544)

17. A. A student radiologic technologist under age 18 should maintain exposure levels below 100 mrem/yr. (Ref. 6, p. 540)

18. B. The MPD categories for one year are: 5 rem/yr = eye lens and gonads; 15 rem/yr = thyroid, lungs, and skin; 30 rem/yr = forearms; 75 rem/yr = hands and feet. (Ref. 29, p. 544)

19. D. Lowest patient dosage = low mAs, high kV, and high filtration. (Ref. 29, p. 563)

20. C. The 13-week MPD for the forearms is 10 rem. (Ref. 29, p. 544)

21. B. The skin erythema dose required to affect 50% of persons so irradiated (SED 50) is about 600 rads (66 Gy). (Ref. 6, p. 502)

22. C. The roentgen is equal to the radiation intensity that will create 2.08×10^9 ion pairs in a cubic centimeter of air; that is, $1 \text{ R} = 2.08 \times 10^9$ ion pairs per centimeter. (Ref. 6, p. 12)

23. D. A conversion from a 6:1 grid to a 16:1 grid would double the amount of mAs required in order to maintain the same radiographic density. The mAs needed for the 16:1 grid substitution would be 120 mAs. (Ref. 11, p. 144)

24. B. According to the inverse square law, if a change of 40 in to 120 in = 1/9 the intensity; 1/9 of 450 mR = 50 mR. (Ref. 6, p. 64)

25. A. Biological effects usually are related to the radiation absorbed dose and, therefore, the rad or gray are units describing the quantity of radiation received. (Ref. 6, p. 13)

26. B. One rem equals 0.01 Sv; therefore, 5 rem equals 5 × 0.01 = 0.05, or 50 mSv. (Ref. 6, p. 13)

27. C. The rem is the unit of dose equivalent (DE) or occupational exposure. It is used to express the quantity of radiation received by radiation workers. (Ref. 6, p. 14)

28. D. All three values represent the cumulative MPD for occupationally exposed persons over 18 years of age. Students under 18 years of age may not receive more than 100 mrem/yr (1 mSv/yr) during the course of their educational activities. (Ref. 6, p. 540)

29. B. MPD = 5 rem/yr. 5 − 3 = 2 rem. (Ref. 6, p. 540)

30. A. 4 in to 32 in = 8 × distance increase. 8^2 = 64, inverse = 1/64 of original mR. 512 mR ÷ 64 = 8 mR. (Ref. 6, p. 64)

31. C.
$$\frac{20}{x} = \frac{48}{72} = \frac{2^2}{3^2} = \frac{4}{9}$$
$$4x = 180$$
$$x = 45 \text{ R} \quad \text{(Ref. 6, p. 64)}$$

32. B.
$$\frac{600 \text{ mR}}{x \text{ mR}} = \frac{1.0^2}{0.5^2}$$
$$x \text{ mR} = 0.25 \times 600 \text{ mR}; x = 150 \text{ mR}$$
$$150 \text{ mR} \times \frac{20 \text{ min}}{60 \text{ min}} = 50 \text{ mR} \quad \text{(Ref. 6, p. 65)}$$

34 / Radiography

33. B. The greater penetrating ability of higher energy radiation permits a greater quantity of radiation to pass through the body part to reach the film. (Ref. 11, p. 80)

34. D. $\dfrac{I_1}{I_2} = \dfrac{D_2^2}{D_1^2}$ $\dfrac{120}{x} = \dfrac{18}{72} = \dfrac{2^2}{8^2} = \dfrac{4}{64}$

4x = 7,680

x = 1,920 mR   (Ref. 6, p. 65)

35. C. The prefix *milli* means 10^{-3}, so $100 \times 10^{-3} = 0.1$ A. (Ref. 29, p. 29)

36. B. $150 \times 9 = 1,350 \div 4 = 337.5$ mR, or approximately 340 mR. (Ref. 6, p. 65)

37. B. The rad has been used as the unit of absorbed dose. This unit indicates the amount of radiant energy transferred to an irradiated object by any type of ionizing radiation. (Ref. 31, p. 36)

38. C. The eye lens, whole body, and gonads can receive 1.25 rem/13-wk period, or 5 rem/yr. Skin can receive 7.5 rem/13-wk period, or 15 rem/yr. (Ref. 29, p. 544)

39. C. Radiation measuring instruments usually are calibrated in roentgens. The output of x-ray machines is specified in roentgens or sometimes milliroentgens (mR). (Ref. 6, p. 13)

40. D. Use of the rad allows quantitation of the amount of ionizing radiation energy transferred by any type of radiation to any target material, not just air. One rad is equal to 100 ergs/g (10^{-2} Gy). (Ref. 6, p.13)

41. D. MPD for whole-body radiation for persons over 18 years of age must not exceed 5 rem (5,000 mrem). (Ref. 29, p. 544)

42. D. Brain necrosis occurs in the low 5,000-rad level. The other three conditions occur in the 200- to 1,000-rad exposure level. (Ref. 6, p. 468)

43. B. Central nervous system death requires a dose rate of 5,000 rad, with a mean survival time of 0 to 3 days. The clinical signs and symptoms are the same as GI, ataxia, edema, vasculitis, and meningitis. (Ref. 6, p. 496)

44. C.   The rad is the unit of radiation-absorbed dose. Biological effects usually are related to the radiation dose; therefore, the rad is the unit most often used when describing the radiation quality received by a patient or experimental animal. (Ref. 6, p. 13)

45. A.   5(N − 18) MPD formula = 35 − 18 = 17 × 5 = 85 − 10 = 75 R. (Ref. 6, p. 540)

46. D.   MPD for the skin is 15 rem in any given year, which is three times MPD for whole-body occupational exposure. (Ref. 6, p. 540)

47. A. $\dfrac{I_1}{I_2} = \dfrac{D_2^2}{D_1^2}$ $\dfrac{75}{x} = \dfrac{90^2}{50^2} = \dfrac{81}{25}$

81x = 1,875 x = 23.1 mR   (Ref. 6, p. 63)

48. B.   Radiation quality is the wavelength of the radiation, determined by the kVp. (Ref. 6, p. 174)

49. B.   The MPD for skin is 15 rem/yr, or 15,000 mrem/yr. (Ref. 6, p. 540)

50. B.   The MPD for the fetus in utero from occupational exposure of a pregnant woman is 0.5 rem, or 500 mrem, during the entire period of gestation. (Ref. 31, p. 56)

51. C.   Combined whole-body exposure for occupational workers is 5 rem/yr. (Ref. 31, p. 56)

52. C.   Dose is directly proportional to time spent in radiation. By combining time spent and distance, the dosage will be reduced to 1/2 × 1/4 = 1/8 of the original. (Ref. 6, p. 536)

53. A.   The radiographer normally stands back or behind the radiologist so that their exposure and, therefore, dose will be decreased. (Ref. 6, p. 537)

54. A. $4,000 \div 4\,(2\,\text{HVL}) = 1,000;\ 1,000 \div 4\,(2 \times \text{distance}) = 250$ (Ref. 29, p. 179)

55. C.   A protective curtain or panel of at least 0.15 mm lead equivalent should be positioned between the fluoroscopist and the patient. (Ref. 6, p. 554)

56. C. $\dfrac{40}{x} = \dfrac{36}{72} = \dfrac{1^2}{2^2} = \dfrac{1}{4}$

$x = 160$ mR   (Ref. 6, p. 64)

57. D.   If the radiographer participates in fluoroscopy and wears a protective apron, as recommended, then the personal monitor should be positioned on the collar above the protective apron. Exposure to the collar region is 10 to 20 times greater than that to the trunk of the body beneath the protective lead apron. (Ref. 6, p. 587)

58. B.   Somatic effects include various kinds of damage that appear during the lifetime of an individual exposed to radiation. Thresholds or lower limits have not been established. (Ref. 29, p. 549)

59. C.   Lungs and thyroid yearly MPD is 15 rem; hand, forearms, and feet yearly MPD is 75 rem; but the lens of the eye is 1.25 rem/13 wk, or 5 rem/yr. (Ref. 29, p. 544)

60. B.   The penetrating ability of an x-ray beam is called quality; this quality is identified by the amount of filtration used in the beam. (Ref. 6, p. 175)

61. B.   To reduce exposure to 1/4 the original requires a doubling of the SID. (Ref. 6, p. 65)

62. D.   Lymphocytes, spermatogonia, and erythroblasts are all cell types of high radiosensitivity with endothelial cells being in an intermediate range. (Ref. 6, p. 467)

63. D.   In the new international system of units, the rad is being replaced by the gray, 1 Gy = 100 rad. (Ref. 29, p. 196)

64. A. The lowest mAs and highest kVp will yield the lowest patient dosage. (Ref. 31, p. 141)

65. C. 1 R = 1,000 mR; therefore, 0.2 R is equal to 200 mR. (Ref. 6, p. 12)

66. C. In the high-sensitivity cell types are lymphocytes, spermatogonia, erythroblasts, and intestinal crypt cells. Spermatids are categorized in the intermediate radiosensitivity category. (Ref. 6, p. 467)

67. C. There are five principal types of molecules in the body. The breakdown is: 80% water, 15% protein, 2% lipids, and 1% each of carbohydrates, nucleic acid, and other substances. (Ref. 6, p. 458)

68. A. The gastrointestinal syndrome occurs between 1,000 and 5,000 rad dosage. (Ref. 6, p. 497)

69. A. The cells of the ovaries respond differently (genetic) to radiation because of differences in progression of the germ cells from the stem cell phase to the mature cell. (Ref. 6, p. 533)

70. A. The early effects of radiation on humans under the acute radiation syndrome include hematologic, gastrointestinal, and central nervous system syndromes. (Ref. 6, p. 496)

71. A. Late or delayed radiation effects on humans can cause leukemia, other malignant diseases, local tissue damage, lifespan shortening, and genetic damage. Prominent cancers can develop in bone, lung, thyroid, and breasts. (Ref. 6, p. 524)

72. D. Somatic effects relate to cells of the body other than the oogonium of the female and the spermatogonium of the male. (Ref. 31, p. 104)

73. C. The pelvis delivers an estimated dose of 100 mrad, extremity 10 mrad, skull 50 mrad and abdomen 80 mrad. (Ref. 31, p. 8)

74. A. A low radiosensitivity exists for muscle cells, nerve cells, and chondrocytes. (Ref. 6, p. 467)

75. A. The lumbar spine is estimated to deliver 700 mrad, IVP 600 mrad, upper GI 150 mrad, and pelvis 210 mrad. (Ref. 31, p. 9)

76. D. Under the summary of acute radiation lethality, the gastrointestinal stage occurs in the dose range of 1,000 to 5,000 rad, with a mean survival time of 4 to 10 days. (Ref. 6, p. 497)

77. B. Lymphocytes and spermatogonia are high and fibroblasts are of intermediate radiosensitivity. (Ref. 6, p. 467)

78. C. Both DNA and RNA are the two principle nucleic acids important to human metabolism. (Ref. 6, p. 460)

79. A. Alpha particles do not penetrate matter for any appreciable depth because of their strong ionizing ability. (Ref. 29, p. 478)

80. A. The older adult relative must be provided with protective apparel positioned away from the primary beam. Radiology personnel should never be used to hold patients. (Ref. 6, p. 589)

81. A. $\dfrac{240 \text{ mR/hr}}{60 \text{ mR/hr}} = 4 \text{ mR/min} \times 4 \text{ min} = 16 \text{ mR}$
(Ref. 6, p. 65)

82. B. The hematologic stage occurs from a dose of 200 to 1,000 rad with a mean survival time of 10 to 60 days. (Ref. 6, p. 497)

83. A. Lymphocytes are categorized as being highly radiosensitive. Endothelial cells and fibroblasts are in the intermediate range, and chondrocytes have a low radiosensitivity. (Ref. 6, p. 467)

84. A. According to estimated average bone marrow doses, a lumbar spine examination yields 400 mrad, abdomen 80 mrad, pelvis 100 mrad, and skull 50 mrad. (Ref. 31, p. 68)

85. B. A pregnant technologist should be removed from fluoroscopy, special procedures, and portable work, for these activities have been shown to result in the bulk of departmental exposure. (Ref. 6, p. 543)

86. D. The hematopoietic or "bone marrow syndrome" occurs when a human receives whole-body doses of ionizing radiation ranging from 1 to 10 Gy (100 to 1,000 rad). (Ref. 31, p. 105)

87. B. If 60 mAs produces 300 mR, then 60 mAs × 5mR/mAs would equal 300 mR. (Ref. 6, p. 22)

88. A. Radiation exposure during the first month of pregnancy is critical since the fetus is extremely sensitive to radiation exposure at this time. The ten-day rule should be followed to decrease this risk. (Ref. 6, p. 547)

89. B. Radiation-induced leukemia is a delayed, linear, nonthreshold response with a latent period of 4 to 7 years, and an at-risk period of approximately 20 years. (Ref. 9, p. 373)

90. B. The blood-forming organs, especially bone marrow, have a high radiosensitivity. Lymphoid and gonadal tissues are also at a high level of radiosensitivity. (Ref. 6, p. 468)

91. B. The inherent filtration of a general purpose x-ray tube is usually about 0.5 mm Al equivalent. This can vary by many manufacturers. With age, this inherent filtration tends to increase. Some tube windows may be made of beryllium rather than glass, and have inherent filtrations of approximately 0.1 mm Al. (Ref. 6, p. 179)

92. D. According to the law of Bergonie and Tribondeau, radiosensitivity is greatest in the cells that are young and have high levels of metabolic activity. (Ref. 6, p. 468)

93. B. In the category of high radiosensitivity are lymphocytes, spermatogonia, erythroblasts, and intestinal crypt cells. (Ref. 6, p. 467)

94. C. The relative risk of childhood leukemia following irradiation in utero by trimesters is: first = 8.3; second = 1.5; third = 1.4, with a marked decrease after birth. (Ref. 6, p. 530)

95. C. Soft tissue radiography requires low kV levels which increase patient absorption. A prime example of soft-tissue high dosage radiography is mammography. (Ref. 6, p. 330)

96. C. Attenuation levels at 75 kV for lead aprons are 0.25 = 66%, 0.50 = 88%, and 1.0 = 99%. (Ref. 6, p. 589)

97. B. Each lipid molecule is composed of one molecule of glycerol and three molecules of fatty acid. (Ref. 6, p. 459)

98. C. Epilation is a response of the skin to radiation exposure. For many years, soft rays (10 to 20 kV) and Grenz rays caused this when used in treatment of skin diseases and ringworm. (Ref. 6, p. 502)

99. A. Biologic tissue is more sensitive to radiation when irradiated in the oxygenated or aerobic state than when irradiated under anoxic or hypoxic conditions. (Ref. 6, p. 470)

100. C. Leakage radiation for the average radiographic tube shall not exceed an average value of 100 mR/hr at 1 m, the required shielding being about 1.5 mm (about 1/16 in) lead. (Ref. 29, p. 552)

101. D. Twelve pulse, three-phase power results in only 3.5% ripple, and the voltage supplied to the x-ray tube stays above 96.5%. (Ref. 6, p. 105)

102. A. For a given phosphor, the thicker the active layer, the greater the speed. Larger crystals impart greater speed because they receive more x-ray photons and scatter less light. (Ref. 29, p. 300)

103. A. Screens with a speed of 200 require 50% less exposure than screens with a speed of 100 for equal radiographic density. With the exposure time reduced, less milliamperage is required. (Ref. 29, p. 299)

104. D. Silver bromide and silver iodide are examples of silver halides. (Ref. 29, p. 288)

105. B. Estimated dosages are 120 mR femur, 980 mR dorsal and cervical spine, 1,320 barium enema, and 670 for an abdomen KUB film. (Ref. 29, p. 561)

106. B. Bone marrow = 4.2%; skin = 2.9%; subcutaneous tissue = 5.8%; and blood = 7.7%. (Ref. 6, p. 467)

107. A. The slowest-speed screen would yield the least amount of mottle and would, therefore, produce the best possible ultra-screen detail. (Ref. 29, p. 305)

108. B. Some rare-earth phosphors include barium strontium sulfate, barium fluorochloride, gadolinium, lanthanum, and terbium. (Ref. 29, p. 300)

109. C. Some rare-earth screens made of gadolinium and lanthanum emit light mainly in the green region of the spectrum. Others can emit violet and blue light. (Ref. 20, p. 300)

110. C. A combination of fast-speed film and high-speed screens can lower the exposure considerably. (Ref. 29, p. 299)

111. A. Modern safety film has a base of about 0.2 mm (7 mils or 0.007 in) thick. (Ref. 29, p. 287)

112. D. A radiograph of an extremity may require 100 mA, 1/30 sec, 54 kV with medium-speed screens. With a cardboard holder, the technique required would be approximately 100 mAs at 52 kV. Therefore, from 20 to 30 times more exposure is required. (Ref. 29, p. 291)

113. C. Lithium fluoride is the most widely used TLD material. It has an effective atomic number of 8.2 and, therefore, has photon absorption properties similar to that of soft tissue. (Ref. 6, p. 569)

114. D. The radiation that has passed through the various thicknesses, types, and densities of tissue interposed between the tube and the film is called remnant or exit radiation. (Ref. 29, p. 321)

115. B. The TLD can measure doses as low as 10 mrad with modest accuracy, and have particular advantage over other monitoring devices. (Ref. 6, p. 569)

116. B. The special derived SI unit for dose equivalent is the sievert (Sv). This has the same basic units as absorbed dose in man. (Ref. 26, p. 51)

117. D. In addition to these advantages, the TLD has accuracy to ±5%,

42 / Radiography

is relatively inexpensive, and is small enough to be incorporated into jewelry. (Ref. 29, p. 548)

118. B. Coherent or unmodified scattering occurs when a very low energy x-ray photon interacts with a relatively bound orbital electron and sets it into vibration. (Ref. 29, p. 189)

119. A. The incident photon will give up all its energy to the atom; in other words, the photon is truly absorbed and disappears during the interaction. (Ref. 29, p. 187)

120. B. Absorption of radiation accompanies the various types of interactions between its photons and the atoms in the irradiated material. Photoelectric interaction with true absorption predominates, with radiation energy up to about 140 kVp. (Ref. 29, p. 200)

121. A. Scattered radiation refers to those x-ray photons that have undergone a change in direction after interacting with atoms. (Ref. 29, p. 184)

122. C. Pair production occurs when a megavoltage photon with energy of at least 1.02 meV splits into a positron and negatron. (Ref. 29, p. 191)

123. B. Compton scattering poses a danger to radiation workers, especially in fluoroscopy. (Ref. 6, p. 159)

124. D. When a very low energy x-ray photon interacts with a relatively bound orbital electron, it sets the electron into a vibration. This unmodified scattering occurs in energy levels below the range useful in clinical radiology. (Ref. 29, p. 189)

125. B. The Compton electron acquires a certain amount of kinetic energy which must be subtracted from the energy of the entering photon. (Ref. 29, p. 189)

126. B. The TLD can measure doses as low as 10 mrad (0.1 mGy), and at doses exceeding 10 rad (100 mGy), accuracy is better than ±5%. (Ref. 29, p. 569)

127. C. If an incident (entering) photon of sufficient energy encounters a loosely bound outer shell electron, it may dislodge the electron and proceed in a different direction. (Ref. 29, p. 189)

128. B. These filters measure the approximate energy of the radiation reaching the monitoring device. (Ref. 31, p. 188)

129. A. Some thermoluminescent materials were able to show that exposure to ionizing radiation caused them to glow. (Ref. 6, p. 569)

130. B. A lead apron with 0.5 mm lead equivalent provides 88% attenuation at 75 kV, which is sufficient. (Ref. 6, p. 543)

131. B. Secondary radiation is produced when high-energy outer shell electrons fill a space in a lower energy orbit, and the energy difference is given off as secondary (characteristic) radiation. (Ref. 29, p. 184)

132. B. A serious problem associated with exposure to radiation is the genetic hazard. Whenever possible, we must shield the gonads (ovaries and testicles) during diagnostic procedures. (Ref. 29, p. 551)

133. C. Blood comprises 7.7% of total body composition; organs compose 12.4%. (Ref. 6, p. 467)

134. A. In mitosis, the division phase is characterized by four subphases: prophase, metaphase, anaphase, and telophase. (Ref. 6, p. 465)

135. A. High radiosensitivity exists for the following cell types: lymphocytes, spermatogonia, erythroblasts, and intestinal crypt cells. (Ref. 6, p. 467)

136. B. Clinical signs and symptoms of the gastrointestinal syndrome are the same as hematologic, electrolyte imbalance, lethargy, fatigue, and shock. (Ref. 6, p. 497)

137. B. The prodromal stage of up to 100 rad can cause nausea, diarrhea, and vomiting. (Ref. 6, p. 497)

138. B. There are five principal types of molecules in the body: water,

44 / Radiography

80%; protein, 15%; lipids, 2%; carbohydrates, 1%; and nucleic acid, 1%. (Ref. 6, p. 458)

139. D. Chondrocytes have a low radiosensitivity. (Ref. 6, p. 467)

140. C. Hormones are produced and secreted by the endocrine glands: the pituitary, adrenal, thyroid, parathyroid, pancreas, and gonads. (Ref. 6, p. 459)

141. B. Atomic composition shows hydrogen, 60%; oxygen, 25.7%, carbon, 10.7%; nitrogen, 2.4%; calcium, 0.2%; phosphorus, 0.1%; sulfur, 0.1%; and trace elements, 0.8%. (Ref. 6, p. 457)

142. A. The stem cells of the ovaries are the oogonia; they multiply in number only during fetal life. (Ref. 6, p. 502)

143. B. In 1953, Watson and Crisk described the molecular structure of DNA, the genetic substance of the cell. (Ref. 6, p. 460)

144. D. Erythroblasts have a high radiosensitivity. (Ref. 6, p. 467)

145. A. The stromal part is composed of connective tissue and vasculature that provides structure to the organ. (Ref. 6, p. 468)

146. B. Every x-ray tube must be contained within a protective housing that reduces the leakage radiation to less than 100 mR/hr at a 1-m distance. (Ref. 6, p. 109)

147. D. The film badge can be used to monitor x-rays, gamma rays, and all but very low beta radiation in a reliable manner. (Ref. 31, p. 190)

148. D. Four inches of concrete is equivalent to 1/16 in of lead, and is usually used instead of lead for wall barriers. (Ref. 6, p. 555)

149. A. The MPD equivalent for the eye lens during a 13-week period is 1.25 rem. (Ref. 29, p. 544)

150. C. The hands and feet can receive 25 rem in a 13-week period; but the forearms can receive only 10 rem. (Ref. 29, p. 544)

2 Equipment Operation and Maintenance

The major subject areas covered in equipment operation and maintenance include the following.

1. Radiography equipment, including the control panel, x-ray tubes, various generation systems, automatic exposure control devices, and operational guidelines.
2. Production and properties of x-ray, generation and rectification, x-ray circuitry, single- and three-phase generation.
3. Types of equipment, including fluoroscopic units, portable machines, and accessories.
4. Maintenance of various radiographic units, various performance tests for calibration, timer accuracy, focal spot size, and various tests to check protective leaded accessories.
5. Various beam restriction devices, corrective action for malfunctions, application and maintenance of various image receptors.
6. Specialized equipment operation and maintenance.

DIRECTIONS (Questions 151–250): Each of the questions or incomplete statements below is followed by four suggested answers or completions. Select the **one** that is best in each case.

---

151. When electrons strike the anode of an x-ray tube, **MOST** of their energy is converted to heat. The percentage of energy converted to x-ray is in the range of
    A. 0.05%
    B. 0.2%
    C. 10.0%
    D. 99.8%

152. Radiation from the tube housing other than the primary beam is called
    A. remnant
    B. secondary
    C. Compton
    D. leakage

153. The focal spot that is projected toward the film is called the
    A. actual
    B. effective
    C. linear
    D. double

154. The stream of electrons in an x-ray tube is focused by the
    A. line-focus principle
    B. potential difference
    C. molybdenum collar around the filament
    D. tilted target

155. If a portable unit has an incoming voltage of 220 V and only 1/4 of the turns of the autotransformer are being used, the voltage tapped off and sent to the high-voltage transformer would be
    A. 25 V
    B. 55 V
    C. 220 V
    D. 440 V

156. The anode cooling chart plots
    A. kV versus mA versus time
    B. heat units produced versus time
    C. heat units produced versus number of exposures
    D. anode temperature versus residual space charge

157. Which of the following is **MOST** likely to damage the x-ray tube?
    A. Excessive vibration
    B. Poor insulation
    C. Excessive anode speed
    D. High mAs values

158. The heat storage capacity of the anode of a diagnostic tube is
    A. 50,000 to 60,000 HU
    B. 70,000 to 400,000 HU
    C. 500,000 to 750,000 HU
    D. over 1,000,000 HU

159. The line focus principle concerns the
    A. angling of the actual focal area on the anode to produce a smaller effective focal spot
    B. thermionic emission of electrons on the cathode
    C. partial absorption of x-rays on the angled part of the anode
    D. maintenance of a constant voltage supply by the line voltage compensator

160. The size of the effective focal spot depends on the
    A. cathode connections
    B. angle of the anode
    C. rotor motor
    D. target material

161. The smallest possible effective focal spot is accomplished by using
    A. low-kV and high-mA settings
    B. low-mA and high-kV settings
    C. high-mA and high-kV settings
    D. low-mA and low-kV settings

162. The size of the focal spot is primarily controlled by the size of the
   A. focusing cup
   B. target size
   C. anode angle
   D. tungsten filament

163. Generally speaking, a large focal spot will be found at which of the mA values?
   A. Under 25 mA
   B. 25 to 50 mA
   C. 200 to 500 mA
   D. Filaments controlling mA from 0.5 to 1.0 mm

164. An excessive tube vibration causes
   A. magnification of the image
   B. diminished sharpness of the image
   C. fluctuation in kilovoltage
   D. excessive density

165. Which of the following would **NOT** be essential in the production of x-radiation?
   A. A source of electrons
   B. Electrons flowing from the anode to the cathode
   C. A high potential difference across the tube
   D. A sudden stoppage of the electrons

166. In modern rotating anode tubes, the target area is coated with
   A. tungsten copper alloy
   B. molybdenum magnesium alloy
   C. tungsten rhenium alloy
   D. pure copper to dissipate heat

167. A tube with a smaller focal spot will
   A. require more mAs
   B. have less penumbra
   C. demonstrate better contrast
   D. have more penumbra

168. The material added to the x-ray tube filament to **INCREASE** its
life and emission efficiency is
   A. rhenium
   B. molybdenum
   C. thorium
   D. copper

169. The focusing cup surrounds the
   A. anode
   B. filament
   C. rotor
   D. glass envelope

170. The glass envelope, cooling oil, and target material of the x-ray tube
are all examples of
   A. added filtration
   B. inherent filtration
   C. total filtration
   D. beam restrictors

171. **MOST** radiologic tube failures are due to
   A. loss of tube vacuum
   B. burning the filament
   C. insufficient current
   D. damage to the target

172. When the mA is changed from a large to a small focal spot, which
of the following is **TRUE**?
   A. Penumbra will decrease
   B. Inverse square law should be applied
   C. Penetrating power increases
   D. Density will double

173. Which of the following devices is used to alter filament, current,
and voltage?
   A. Line voltage compensator
   B. Choke coil
   C. Autotransformer
   D. Valve tube

174. Filament current is measured in
  A. ohms
  B. milliamperes
  C. amperes
  D. kilovolts

175. The purpose of the cathode focusing cup is to
  A. alter filament size
  B. group the electrons for their passage to the anode
  C. regulate radiographic quality
  D. change the beam's intensity

176. The source of electrons in a rotating anode tube is the
  A. rotor
  B. anode
  C. filament
  D. focal track

177. With prolonged use, the temperature of the filament in the x-ray tube tends to
  A. rise
  B. fall
  C. stabilize
  D. fluctuate

178. If the anode heel effect is measured with a 7° anode angle at 100 cm and is found to cover a 25-cm distance, then a 20° anode angle at the same TFD would cover approximately
  A. three times as much, or 75 cm
  B. 1/3 as much, or 8.3 cm
  C. nine times as much, or 225 cm
  D. the same, or 25 cm

179. The anode in a rotating tube is composed of
  A. tungsten embedded in copper
  B. molybdenum and magnesium
  C. mushroon-shaped disc of tungsten
  D. pyrex leaded glass

180. The area in the x-ray tube that is bombarded by the electron stream is called the
  A. filament
  B. actual focal spot
  C. effective focal spot
  D. focus cup

181. The formula that calculates the heat units produced by a three-phase six-pulse tube is
  A. $kV \times mA \times time$
  B. $kV \times mA \times time \times 0.60$
  C. $kV \times mA \times time \times 1.35$
  D. $kV \times mA \times time \times 1.41$

182. What part of the x-ray tube must be able to accumulate, store, and discharge great quantities of heat?
  A. Filament
  B. Focusing cup
  C. Cathode
  D. Anode

183. The target material of an x-ray tube must have a high
  1. electrical resistance
  2. melting point
  3. atomic number
  A. 1 and 2 only
  B. 1 and 3 only
  C. 2 and 3 only
  D. 1, 2, and 3

184. Increasing the potential difference between the cathode and anode will result in an **INCREASE** in the
  1. number of x-rays
  2. energy of the x-rays
  3. frequency of the x-rays
  A. 1 and 2 only
  B. 2 and 3 only
  C. 1 and 3 only
  D. 1, 2, and 3

185. The beveled edge around the rotating anode disc on which heat from the electron stream is distributed is called the

   A. focal spot
   B. effective focus
   C. actual focus
   D. focal track

186. Which of the following may happen as a result of the application of excessive heat to the anode of an x-ray tube?

   1. Pitting and cracking of the anode
   2. Tungsten coating on glass envelope
   3. Reduced x-ray output
   A. 1 and 2 only
   B. 1 and 3 only
   C. 2 and 3 only
   D. 1, 2, and 3

187. How many watts are produced by a current of 50 A and 10 V?

   A. 40
   B. 60
   C. 500
   D. 5,000

188. The atomic numbers (z) and melting points (mp) of four possible metals for an x-ray tube target are listed below. The **BEST** selection for a given tube is

   A. $z = 74$, $mp = 3370\ °C$
   B. $z = 6$, $mp = 3500\ °C$
   C. $z = 79$, $= mp = 1063\ °C$
   D. $z = 78$, $mp = 1770\ °C$

189. The range of wavelengths in angstroms associated with diagnostic radiology is

   A. 0.01 to 0.5
   B. 0.1 to 0.5
   C. 1.0 to 5.0
   D. 10.0 to 50.0

190. Which of the following is **NOT** a property of x-rays?
   A. Highly penetrating, invisible rays
   B. Electrically neutral
   C. Monoenergetic wavelengths
   D. Travel in straight lines

191. Which of the following changes occurs when the kV is changed from 65 to 80?
   A. Amount of photons increases
   B. Frequency increases
   C. Speed decreases
   D. Scatter radiation decreases

192. If the distance of two magnets is cut in half, the force of attraction or repulsion would be
   A. one-fourth of the original intensity
   B. four times as much
   C. two times as much
   D. one-half of the original intensity

193. All x-ray photons travel at a velocity of
   A. 8×10^3 m/sec
   B. 3×10^{10} m/sec
   C. 3×10^8 m/sec
   D. 10×3^8 m/sec

194. Which of the following statements is **FALSE**?
   A. Electric charges reside on external surfaces
   B. Unlike charges attract and like charges repel
   C. Only neutrons can move in solid conductors
   D. If the strength of unlike magnets is doubled, then the force of attraction is four times as much

195. The radiologic image is composed mainly of
   A. primary radiation
   B. secondary radiation
   C. scattered radiation
   D. remnant radiation

196. Heating the x-ray tube's filament to incandescence will produce
1. thermionic emission
2. free electrons
3. space charge

   A. 1 and 2 only
   B. 1 and 3 only
   C. 2 and 3 only
   D. 1, 2, and 3

197. The x-ray beam that emerges from the target of an x-ray tube consists of
   A. remnant and exit radiations
   B. alpha and beta radiations
   C. brems and characteristic radiations
   D. scattered and secondary radiations

198. A highly penetrating x-ray beam consists of rays which, on the average, have a
1. high energy
2. short wavelength
3. high frequency

   A. 1 and 2 only
   B. 1 and 3 only
   C. 2 and 3 only
   D. 1, 2, and 3

199. A transformer with more turns in its secondary coil than in its primary coil would be expected to
   A. increase the voltage and decrease the amperage
   B. increase the voltage and the amperage
   C. decrease the voltage and increase the amperage
   D. decrease the voltage and the amperage

200. Which of the following are valid reasons for a transformer to be submerged in a tank filled with a special oil?
1. To maximize electrical insulation
2. To minimize rust and oxidation
3. To help cool the transformer
   A. 1 and 2 only
   B. 1 and 3 only
   C. 2 and 3 only
   D. 1, 2, and 3

201. An individual x-ray may be regarded as a tiny bit of energy called a
1. photon
2. quantum
3. angstrom
   A. 1 and 2 only
   B. 1 and 3 only
   C. 2 and 3 only
   D. 1, 2, and 3

202. How many volts are required to move a current of 60 A across a circuit having a resistance of 2 Ω?
   A. 15
   B. 30
   C. 60
   D. 120

203. Which of the following has the longest wavelength?
   A. Infrared
   B. Radio
   C. Ultraviolet
   D. Gamma

204. Which of the following techniques would produce the greatest number of HU?
   A. 200 mA, 1/40 sec, 90 kV, one-half wave generator
   B. 500 mA, 1/20 sec, 85 kV, three-phase generator
   C. 400 mA, 1/30 sec, 80 kV, full-wave generator
   D. 300 mA, 1/60 sec, 80 kV, three-phase generator

205. Which of the following can occur if the anode thermal capacity of the tube is exceeded?
1. Warping of the anode
2. Gas emission
3. Melting of the anode
A. 1 and 2 only
B. 1 and 3 only
C. 2 and 3 only
D. 1, 2, and 3

206. From which electron shell is the highest energy-characteristic x-ray emitted?
A. K
B. L
C. M
D. N

207. An x-ray beam that is composed of individual rays with many different wavelengths is said to be
1. heterogeneous
2. polyenergetic
3. homogenous
A. 1 and 2 only
B. 1 and 3 only
C. 2 and 3 only
D. 1, 2, and 3

208. The size of the focal spot has little to do with detail when SID is greater than
A. 20 in
B. 36 in
C. 40 in
D. 72 in

209. A 1/20 sec exposure is made with a self-rectified generator. How many dots will be demonstrated on the film by the spinning top test?
A. 3
B. 6
C. 8
D. 10

210. A transformer has 1,000 turns in the primary coil and 10,000 turns in the secondary. What is the voltage in the secondary coil if there are 220 V applied to the primary coil?
A. 22 V
B. 220 V
C. 2,200 V
D. 22 kV

211. If the heat storage capacity of an x-ray tube is 32,000 BTU, what would be the maximum number of exposures allowed using the following factors: 300 mA; 1/20 sec; 70 kV?
A. 30
B. 34
C. 40
D. 60

212. How many heat units would be produced in a single-phase operation utilizing a radiographic technique of 200 mA, 1/2 sec, 60 kV, at a 40-in FFD?
A. 600 HU
B. 2,400 HU
C. 6,000 HU
D. 24,000 HU

213. The type of current required for transformer operation is
A. direct
B. three-phase
C. single-phase
D. alternating

214. Which of the following is used in calibrating x-ray equipment?
A. Spinning top
B. Penetrometer
C. Dosimeter
D. Densitometer

215. Which of the following devices can operate on either direct or alternating current?
A. Choke coil
B. Autotransformer
C. Rheostat
D. X-ray tube

216. A synchronous motor could be used in an x-ray circuit as a/an
A. target rotor
B. ammeter
C. timer
D. current regulator

217. Which of the following would **NOT** be found in the primary (low voltage) side of a x-ray circuit?
A. Autotransformer
B. Timer
C. Exposure switch
D. Solid-state rectifier

218. The **MOST** accurate timer for exposures under 1/10 sec is
A. mechanical
B. synchronous timer
C. electronic impulse timer
D. motor-driven impulse

219. If the mAs was set for 150, but only 75 registered on the meter during the exposure, it could be an indication that
A. the tube housing is leaking
B. a valve tube is burned out
C. the bucky button is not pushed in
D. the tube is not on center lock

220. The heat units for a single-phase rectified unit is 3,000. What would be the heat units for a three-phase, 12-pulse rectified unit using the same factors?
  A. 3,000
  B. 3,750
  C. 4,230
  D. 4,430

221. The device that terminates the exposure when proper radiographic density is obtained is the
  A. rheostat
  B. automatic exposure control
  C. autotransformer
  D. synchronous timer

222. Rectification is a process that changes
  A. pulsating direct current (DC) to alternating current (AC)
  B. alternating current to pulsating direct current
  C. alternating current to direct current
  D. pulsating direct to pulsating alternating current

223. The turns ratio of a high-voltage transformer is 800:1; the supply voltage is peaked at 120 V. What is the secondary voltage supplied to the x-ray tube?
  A. 96 kV
  B. 92 kV
  C. 192 V
  D. 196 V

224. Where are rectifiers located in the x-ray circuit?
  A. Between the high-voltage transformer and the x-ray tube
  B. To the left of the high-voltage transformer
  C. Between the valve tubes and the autotransformer
  D. Before the autotransformer

225. How many pulses would be demonstrated on a radiographic film when utilizing the spinning-top technique and using an exposure time of 1/15 sec on a full-wave rectified unit?
   A. 9
   B. 18
   C. 22
   D. 36

226. An autotransformer functions as a
   A. line voltage compensator
   B. rectifier
   C. kilovolt selector
   D. filament transformer

227. An excessive amount of electrons at one end of a conductor and a deficiency at the other end is known as
   A. space charge
   B. resistance
   C. potential difference
   D. impedance

228. Which device in the filament circuit is operated when the filament control knob is manipulated?
   A. Autotransformer
   B. Valve tubes
   C. Choke coil
   D. Prereading kilovolt meter

229. If we applied 240 V across a resistance of 12 Ω, the resultant current in amps would be
   A. 0.5
   B. 20
   C. 200
   D. 252

230. The current that passes through the high-voltage transformer toward the rectifier is called
   A. alternating current
   B. direct current
   C. pulsating direct current
   D. eddy loss current

231. How much current would be produced when utilizing a pressure of 220 V applied across 5 Ω?
   A. 2.25 A
   B. 44 A
   C. 225 A
   D. 1,100 A

232. If a 10-Ω and a 5-Ω resistor are placed in parallel in a circuit carrying 120 V, the current in the circuit would be
   A. 8 A
   B. 36.3 A
   C. 45.0 A
   D. 80 A

233. Which of the following materials has a high permeability and a low retentivity?
   A. Cobalt
   B. Plastic
   C. Soft iron
   D. Glass

234. A helix carrying current with a soft iron core is a/an
   A. resistant circuit
   B. electromagnet
   C. double helix
   D. rectifier

235. Alternating current is employed much more frequently than direct current. Which of the following is a major reason?
  A. AC is easier to produce
  B. Transformers will only operate on AC
  C. The timing circuit depends on AC
  D. Valve tubes can only operate on AC

236. Which statement regarding Ohm's law is **INCORRECT**?
  A. $\dfrac{V}{I} = R$
  B. $I \times R = V$
  C. $\dfrac{V}{R} = I$
  D. $\dfrac{R}{I} = V$

237. Hysteresis can be minimized by the use of
  A. copper conductors
  B. plastic insulators
  C. rectifiers
  D. silicone steel

238. The unit of capacitance is the
  A. joule
  B. farad
  C. coulomb
  D. watt

239. Modern electronic timers are able to provide accurate exposure times down to
  A. 1/20 sec
  B. 1/16 sec
  C. 1/120 sec
  D. 1/1000 sec

240. A particular transformer is constructed so that there are 100 turns in the primary coil and 100,000 turns in the secondary coil. If the input is 120 V, what is the output voltage going to be?
A. 1.2 V
B. 12 V
C. 12,000 V
D. 120,000 V

241. Three-phase generators operate on three single-phase currents that are out of step with each other by
A. one-quarter cycle, or 90°
B. one-third cycle, or 120°
C. one-half cycle, or 180°
D. one full cycle, or 360°

242. Which of the following terms is used to describe materials that offer tremendous resistance to the flow of electricity?
1. Conductors
2. Insulators
3. Dielectrics
A. 1 and 2 only
B. 1 and 3 only
C. 2 and 3 only
D. 1, 2, and 3

243. A radiographic technique of 200 mA at 1.5 sec and 105 kVp taken on a single-phase, full-wave, rectified unit would produce how many HU?
A. 25,550
B. 31,500
C. 36,000
D. 57,000

244. What is the maximum number of exposures that can safely be made at 200 mA, 90 kV, and 1.5 sec on a single-phase machine with a heat storage capacity of 200,000 HU?
   A. 5
   B. 7
   C. 9
   D. 12

245. Which of the following calculations for determining heat units is CORRECT for a technique of 100 mA, 1 sec, and 80 kVp?
   1. Single-phase (full-wave rectification) = 8,000 HU
   2. Three-phase (six-pulse rectification) = 10,800 HU
   3. Three-phase (12-pulse rectification) = 11,280 HU
   A. 1 and 2 only
   B. 1 and 3 only
   C. 2 and 3 only
   D. 1, 2, and 3

246. How many HU would be eliminated if a radiographic technique of 100 mA, 1 sec, and 85 kV (which is 8,500 HU) were changed to 100 mA, 1/2 sec, and 95 kV?
   A. 3,750 HU
   B. 4,750 HU
   C. 9,500 HU
   D. 13,250 HU

247. What would be the difference in the amount of heat units produced by a single-phase, full-wave rectified unit and by a three-phase, six-pulse rectified unit if a technique of 100 mA, 1 sec, 80 kVp were used by both units?
   A. An increase of 3,280 HU
   B. An increase of 2,800 HU
   C. A decrease of 480 HU
   D. No change in HU totals

248. A circuit with a resistance of 550 Ω, a voltage of 275 V, and a current of 5 A will have a total wattage of
   A. 335 W
   B. 550 W
   C. 1,375 W
   D. 2,750 W

249. A lateral skull tomogram requires 50 mA for 3 sec at 75 kV on a single-phase unit. How many heat units are generated by five exposures?
   A. 9,750
   B. 10,550
   C. 11,250
   D. 56,250

250. An **INCREASE** in EMF in an x-ray tube will affect the
   A. cathode temperature
   B. quality of the beam
   C. quantity of the beam
   D. number of valve tubes utilized

Explanatory Answers

151. B. When the electrons comprising the tube current slam into the anode, more than 99% of their kinetic energy is converted into heat. (Ref. 6, p. 140)

152. D. A properly designed protective housing reduces the level of leakage radiation to less than 100 mR/h at 1 m. (Ref. 6, p. 109)

153. B. The effective target area or effective focal spot size is the area projected onto the patient and the film. (Ref. 6, p. 117)

154. C. The molybdenum collar around the filament carries a negative charge and prevents electrons from scattering backward by repelling them. (Ref. 6, p. 111)

155. B. $220 \div 4 = 55$ volts per turn. (Ref. 29, p. 137)

156. B. The anode cooling curve plots maximum heat units on a graph that shows heat units stored in the anode on a vertical scale and time in minutes plotted horizontally. (Ref. 29, p. 233)

157. D. Excessive mAs values can cause overheating, which will inevitably shorten tube life. (Ref. 29, p. 226)

158. B. The heat storage capacity of the anodes of various diagnostic tubes range from about 70,000 HU to about 400,000 HU, depending on the size of the anode and the cooling method. (Ref. 29, p. 231)

159. A. Angling of the anode face permits a larger actual area on the anode to be bombarded with electrons, thus allowing more heat to be placed on the focal track. (Ref. 6, p. 117)

160. B. By angling the target, one makes the effective area of the target much smaller than the actual area of electron interaction. (Ref. 6, p. 117)

161. B. The low milliampere stations of 25, 50, and 100 are generally employing a small (1.0) focal spot. The kilovoltage can be raised to maintain radiographic density. (Ref. 9, p. 12)

162. D. The tungsten filament is usually about 2 mm in diameter and 1- to 2-cm long. The thermionic emission that takes place is focused towards the focal spot. (Ref. 6, p. 111)

163. C. The large focal spot (2.0) is found in the 200 to 500 mA ranges for most diagnostic units. (Ref. 29, p. 217)

164. B. A seemingly minor vibration in an x-ray tube during an exposure can nullify the effect of the focal spot. (Ref. 8, p. 6)

165. B. To produce x-rays, you are required to separate electrons, produce high-speed electrons, focus them, and stop them at the target. (Ref. 29, p. 162)

166. C. Modern x-ray tubes utilize an anode composition of either solid tungsten or molybdenum coated with a rhenium tungsten alloy. (Ref. 8, p. 3)

167. B. The smaller the effective focal spot, the sharper the radiographic image. As focal spot size decreases, there is a marked increase in image definition. (Ref. 8, p. 3)

168. C. Filaments are usually made of thoriated tungsten, which has a melting point of 3410 °C. (Ref. 6, p. 110)

169. B. A negatively charged concave metal cup behind the filament confines the electrons to a narrow beam and focuses them on a small focal spot on the tungsten target known as the tube focus or focal spot. (Ref. 29, p. 216)

170. B. Inherent filtration of a general purpose tube is usually about 0.5 mm AL equivalent. (Ref. 6, p. 178)

171. B. Filament life is shortened by application of large filament currents (resulting high temperatures). (Ref. 29, p. 235)

172. A. The smaller the effective focal spot, the sharper the radiographic image. (Ref. 8, p. 4)

173. B. The choke coil operates on the principle of self-inductance and creates a decrease in current due to the larger inductance of the circuit. (Ref. 29, p. 141)

174. C. The filament current supplying the filament causes it to become glowing hot or incandescent. It is usually about 3 to 5 A. (Ref. 29, p. 162)

175. B. The metal focusing cup confines the electrons to a narrow beam and focuses them on a small spot on the tungsten target. (Ref. 29, p. 216)

176. C. The filament current, serving to heat the filament and provide a source of electrons within the tube, operates at about 10 V and 3 to 5 A. (Ref. 29, p. 216)

177. A. Loss of metal (tungsten) by evaporation causes the filament to become progressively thinner. It is found that as the tube ages, a progressively lower filament current setting is required for a desired tube milliamperage. (Ref. 29, p. 218)

178. A. The 7° anode covers 25 cm at a 100-cm SID and the 20° anode would cover three times as much area, or 75 cm at the same SID. (Ref. 8, p. 7)

179. C. Rotating anode tubes contain a tungsten disc, shaped somewhat like a mushroom, that rotates approximately 3,300 RPM. (Ref. 8, p. 3)

180. B. The actual focal spot relates to the area bombarded by the electron stream. (Ref. 6, p. 117)

181. C. For three-phase, six-pulse operation, the HU total must be multiplied by the factor 1.35, and for three-phase, 12-pulse, by 1.41. (Ref. 29, p. 231)

182. D. Since more than 99% of the electron's kinetic energy changes to heat at the target, the high melting points of tungsten (3,370 °C) makes it especially suitable as a target metal. (Ref. 29, p. 219)

183. C. The tungsten target has a high melting point of 3,370 °C and an atomic number of 74. (Ref. 29, p. 218)

184. B. An increase in the EMF potential difference, or kVp adjustment, alters beam quality. (Ref. 29, p. 71)

185. D. During rotation, the anode constantly "turns a new face" to the electron beam, so that the heating effect of the beam does not concentrate at one point, as in the stationary anode, but spreads over a large area on the beveled face of the anode called the focal tract. (Ref. 29, p. 223)

186. D. Excessive heat reduces x-ray output because as photons leave the anode, they have to penetrate an uneven surface. Pitting and tungsten coatings can also occur. (Ref. 29, p. 228)

187. C. Watts = V × A. Watts = 50 × 10 = 500. (Ref. 29, p. 86)

188. A. A very high melting point is necessary for an efficient target. Also, the higher the atomic number, the more efficient is the production of x-rays. (Ref. 29, p. 166)

189. B. If we take an energy range for diagnostic radiology, 25 keV to 125 keV, and we use the formula, Wavelength = 12.4/energy in keV, we can calculate the wavelength in angstroms. (Ref. 29, p. 159)

190. C. X-ray wavelengths are polyenergetic or heterogeneous, having a wide span of energies and wavelengths. (Ref. 29, p. 167)

191. B. Frequency is inversely proportional to wavelength. The speed with which the wave travels is equal to the frequency multiplied by the wavelength. (Ref. 29, p. 158)

192. B. The force of attraction (or repulsion) between two magnetic poles varies directly as the strength of the poles and inversely as the square of the distance between them. (Ref. 29, p. 90)

193. C. X-rays travel at the speed of light, 3×10^8 M per sec, or 186,000 miles per sec, in a vacuum. (Ref. 29, p. 167)

194. C. Electrons move in solid conductors. (Ref. 29, p. 57)

195. D. The amount of blackening of a particular area of a radiograph depends on the amount of radiation that has passed through the various thicknesses called remnant or exit radiation. (Ref. 29, p. 321)

196. D. The filament current supplying the filament causes it to become hot or incandescent, with resulting separation of some of its outer orbital electrons. (Ref. 29, p. 162)

197. C. When the fast electron stream enters the tube target, the electrons interact with target atoms, producing x-rays by brems radiation and characteristic radiation. (Ref. 29, p. 163)

198. D. X-rays consist of high-energy, short-wavelength, and high-frequency beams. (Ref. 29, p. 171)

199. A. According to the transformer law, the EMF induced in the secondary coil is to the EMF in the primary coil, as the number of turns in the secondary coil is to the number of turns in the primary coil. (Ref. 29, p. 129)

200. B. In the shell-type transformer, the windings are highly insulated from each other and the entire transformer is submerged in a tank filled with oil for cooling and insulation. (Ref. 29, p. 132)

201. A. Each electromagnetic wave behaves as a bit of energy called a photon or quantum. (Ref. 29, p. 160)

202. D. According to Ohm's law, $V = I \times R$. $V = 60 \times 2 = 120$ V. (Ref. 29, p. 73)

203. B. According to the electromagnetic spectrum, radiowaves equal $3(10)^5$ cm. (Ref. 29, p. 159)

204. B. To calculate the heat units for this exposure, you would multiply $kV \times mA \times sec \times 1.35$ (for three-phase operation). (Ref. 29, p. 231)

205. D. With the production of excessive heat units and not allowing the tube to cool, all three of these conditions can exist. (Ref. 29, p. 228)

206. A. The binding energy is greatest for electrons nearest the atomic nucleus because of the very strong attraction between the negative electrons and the positive protons in the nucleus. (Ref. 29, p. 41)

207. A. X-rays have a wide span of energies and wavelengths, and are classified as polyenergetic or heterogeneous. (Ref. 29, p. 167)

208. D. Image sharpness is enhanced by a small tube focus, short OFD, and long FFD. Blur is minimal from the focal spot size at long FFDs. (Ref. 29, p. 342)

209. A. 60 pulsations divided by 1/20 sec equals 3 dots. (Ref. 29, p. 251)

210. C. $\dfrac{VS}{VP} = \dfrac{NS}{NP}$ $\quad 220 \times 10 = 2{,}200$ V
(Ref. 29, p. 129)

211. A. $300 \times 0.05 = 15$. $15 \times 70 = 1050$. $32{,}000 \div 1050 = 30.48$ exposures. (Ref. 29, p. 231)

212. C. $200\,\text{mA} \times 1/2\,\text{sec} = 100\,\text{mAs}$. $100\,\text{mAs} \times 60\,\text{kVp} = 6{,}000$ HU. (Ref. 29, p. 231)

213. D. An alternating current flowing in the primary coil sets up, in and around it, a magnetic field that varies rapidly in direction and strength. (Ref. 29, p. 130)

214. B. The effects of kilovoltage on contrast are measured by the penetrometer or aluminum step wedge. (Ref. 29, p. 360)

215. C. The rheostat is a device used for voltage control that can operate on either alternating or direct current. (Ref. 29, p. 138)

216. C. The synchronous motor has limited speeds and can be used in electric clocks and synchronous timers. (Ref. 29, p. 122)

217. D. All rectifying systems are located between the secondary coil of the transformer and the x-ray tube. (Ref. 29, p. 270)

218. C. The electronic timer (modern type) provides extremely accurate exposures down to 1 msec (1/1000 sec). (Ref. 29, p. 259)

219. B. Whenever one rectifier diode fails, the system operates as a half-wave rectified unit. (Ref. 29, p. 249)

220. C. kV × mA × sec = 3,000 × 1.41 = 4,230 HU. (Ref. 29, p. 230)

221. B. Automatic control systems utilize an electronic exposure timer that terminates the exposure when the proper radiographic density is obtained. (Ref. 6, p. 305)

222. C. Rectification may be defined as the process of changing alternating current to direct current. (Ref. 29, p. 145)

223. A. Transformer equation $= \dfrac{VS}{VP} = \dfrac{NS}{NP}$
$800 \times 120 = 96,000$, or 96 kV. (Ref. 29, p. 129)

224. A. Rectifiers change current from AC to DC and are located between the step-up transformer and the x-ray tube. (Ref. 29, p. 270)

225. B. $120 \times 0.15 = 18$ pulses. (Ref. 29, p. 249)

226. C. A movable conductor varies the number of turns included in the secondary circuit of the autotransformer, thereby varying its output voltage. Thus, the autotransformer is a kilovolt selector. (Ref. 29, p. 135)

227. C. Potential difference is the difference in electrical potential energy between two points in an electric circuit. (Ref. 29, p. 69)

228. C. Three devices are available for controlling filament current. They are the choke coil, rheostat, and saturable reactor. (Ref. 29, p. 140)

229. B. $240 \text{ V} \div 12 \ \Omega = 20 \text{ A}$. (Ref. 29, p. 79)

230. A. The current approaching the rectifier is still alternating current. (Ref. 29, p. 145)

231. B. 220 V ÷ 5 Ω = 44 A. (Ref. 29, p. 79)

232. A. 5 Ω + 10 Ω = 15 Ω ÷ 120 V = 8 A. (Ref. 29, p. 73)

233. C. Ferromagnetic materials are strongly attracted by a magnet because of their extremely high permeability. Iron, cobalt, and nickel are examples. (Ref. 29, p. 95)

234. B. A helix carrying a current is a solenoid and once the solenoid has an iron core it becomes an electromagnet. (Ref. 29, p. 101)

235. B. A transformer is an electromagnetic device that changes an alternating current from high to low or low to high with minimal loss of energy. (Ref. 29, p. 127)

236. D. $V = I \times R$, according to Ohm's law. (Ref. 29, p. 73)

237. D. Hysteresis loss is a power loss occurring from heat in the transformer core. Laminated silicon steel will minimize the loss. (Ref. 29, p. 134)

238. B. The unit of capacitance is the farad, which is a very large unit. A more practical unit is the microfarad (millionth of a farad). (Ref. 29, p. 85)

239. D. Modern electronic timers provide extremely accurate exposures down to 1 msec (1/1000 of a sec). (Ref. 29, p. 259)

240. D. $\dfrac{VS}{VP} = \dfrac{NS}{NP}$ 120 V × 1,000 = 120,000 V
(Ref. 29, p. 129)

241. B. A three-phase generator operates on three-phase current, which consists of three single-phase currents out of step with each other by one-third cycle, or 120°. (Ref. 29, p. 273)

74 / Radiography

242. C. Insulators or dielectrics oppose the free flow of electric current. (Ref. 29, p. 57)

243. B. 200 mA × 1.5 sec × 105 kV = 31,500 HU. (Ref. 29, p. 230)

244. B. 200 mA × 1.5 sec × 90 kV = 27,000 HU.
200,000 ÷ 27,000 = 7.4 exposures. (Ref. 29, p. 230)

245. D. 80 kV × 100 mA × 1 sec = 8,000 HU
80 kV × 100 mA × 1 sec × 1.35 = 10,800 HU
80 kV × 100 mA × 1 sec × 1.41 = 11,280 HU
(All are calculated correctly.) (Ref. 29, p. 230)

246. A. 8,500 − 4,750 = 3,750 fewer HU produced. (Ref. 29, p. 230)

247. B. Single-phase = 8,000; three-phase = 10,800 = 2,800 additional HU produced. (Ref. 29, p. 230)

248. C. Watts = Amps × Volts. 5 × 275 = 1,375 W. (Ref. 29, p. 86)

249. D. 50 mA × 3 sec × 75 kV = 11,250 × 5 exposures = 56,250 HU. (Ref. 29, p. 230)

250. B. An increase in EMF or kilovoltage gives the x-ray beam more quality. (Ref. 29, p. 159)

3 Image Production and Evaluation

The major subject areas covered in image production and evaluation include the following.

1. Technical factors that affect the radiographic image regarding:
   Density changes involving mAs, distance, kVp, grids, filtration, film and screens, the heel effect, anatomic and pathologic factors.
   Contrast changes involving kVp, collimation, film and screen, grids, filters, anatomic and pathologic factors, as well as short-scale and long-scale contrast concepts.
   Distortion changes involving size distortion by adjustment of the OFD and FFD, and changes involving shape distortion by adjusting the tube, part, film alignment.
   Recorded detail changes involving OFD, FFD, motion, focal spot size, and film screen combinations.
2. Exposure calculations involving:
   a. milliamperage and time (mAs)
   b. kVp: 15% rule
   c. SID, mAs, and distance relationship
   d. grid conversions
   e. film screen combinations and adjustments
   f. anatomic and pathologic factors
3. Film, screens, and grid combinations including film contrast and latitude, anatomical considerations of tissue density, part thickness, and conversion factors for screen and grids.
4. Types of x-ray film, holders, film processing, quality assurance, darkroom design, and factors relating to film storage such as temperature and humidity, radiation and chemical fog, age, safe lights, filters, light leaks, and film bins.

5. Manual and automatic exposure factors relating to phototimers, kVp, mA, and density selections; alignment of part, film, and tube; and changes occurring from anatomic or pathologic conditions.

6. Technique charts, H and D curves, darkroom procedures, technique conversions, calipers, and related radiography accessory equipment.

7. Automatic and manual film processing systems and solutions. Preventive maintenance, artifacts, fog, and testing procedures to ensure film quality.

8. Evaluation of radiographs and corrective action steps for poor quality radiographs.

DIRECTIONS (Questions 251–450): Each of the questions or incomplete statements below is followed by four suggested answers or completions. Select the **one** that is best in each case.

251. The useful range of density for diagnostic radiographic film would range on a densitometer from
   A. 0.03 to 0.1
   B. 0.4 to 2.75
   C. 3.0 to 5.0
   D. 5.5 to 8.0

252. Which of the following is **MOST** opaque?
   A. Muscle
   B. Bone
   C. Cartilage
   D. Solid organs

253. When the technologist is radiographing a PA chest using an air gap technique, which of the following would **NOT** be used?
   A. An erect position
   B. A high-ratio grid
   C. A kV of 120
   D. A 6-in OFD

254. Why is a high kV technique (above 90 kV) recommended for GI studies?
   A. It gives greater detail
   B. It is needed to penetrate the contrast medium
   C. Short-scale contrast is desirable
   D. Less penumbra is present

255. Which of the following changes would have a dramatic effect on radiographic contrast?
   A. change kV from 86 to 82
   B. change focal spot from small to large
   C. change mAs from 100 to 125
   D. change from table top to a 12:1 grid

256. When long wavelength rays interact with thin body parts, the result is
A. short-scale contrast
B. high-scatter production
C. decreased definition
D. long-scale contrast

257. Which of the following affect contrast?
1. Grid ratio
2. OFD
3. Focal spot size
A. 1 and 2 only
B. 1 and 3 only
C. 2 and 3 only
D. 1, 2, and 3

258. Increasing the OFD will magnify the image and **INCREASE** the
A. density
B. definition
C. contrast
D. detail

259. When a film demonstrates long-scale contrast because of over-penetration, the appropriate change to restore a shorter scale of contrast would be
A. increase FFD
B. decrease kV
C. open the collimator more
D. increase mAs 35%

260. A radiograph that demonstrates numerous shades of similar densities is referred to as an image with
A. high contrast
B. low contrast
C. low definition
D. short-scale contrast

261. Which of the following radiographic techniques would produce a radiograph with the longest scale contrast?
  A. 100 mA, 1/4 sec, 65 kVp
  B. 200 mA, 1/2 sec, 85 kVp
  C. 300 mA, 3/10 sec, 75 kVp
  D. 400 mA, 1/5 sec, 70 kVp

262. Which of the following sets of technical factors would produce the shortest scale of contrast?
  A. 100 mA, 0.05 sec, 80 kV, 10:1 grid, small focal spot
  B. 200 mA, 0.10 sec, 60 kV, 12:1 grid, large focal spot
  C. 400 mA, 0.25 sec, 75 kV, 8:1 grid, large focal spot
  D. 600 mA, 0.40 sec, 65 kV, 6:1 grid, small focal spot

263. Which set of technical factors and accessories would produce the shortest scale of contrast?
  A. 12:1 grid, 100 mAs, 90 kV, 14-in × 17-in field size, slow-speed screens
  B. 10:1 grid, 60 mAs, 65 kV, 10-in × 12-in field size, high-speed screens
  C. 8:1 grid, 10 mAs, 70 kV, 14-in × 14-in field size, ultra-detail screens
  D. 6:1 grid, 20 mAs, 80 kV, 12-in × 12-in field size, medium-speed screens

264. Which technique would yield the shortest scale of contrast?
  A. 100 mAs, 60 kV, 10:1 grid, medium-speed screens
  B. 150 mAs, 58 kV, 16:1 grid, high-speed screens
  C. 200 mAs, 62 kV, 12:1 grid, slow-speed screens
  D. 300 mAs, 56 kV, 6:1 grid, medium-speed screens

265. A change of 200 mA, 1/4 sec, 65 kV to 200 mA, 1/8 sec, 75 kV results in a radiograph with
  A. additional density
  B. longer-scale contrast
  C. increased distortion
  D. less penumbra

266. Which of the following sets of technical factors will produce a radiograph with the highest contrast?
   A. 20 mAs, 80 kV, 30-in FFD, 8:1 grid
   B. 15 mAs, 75 kV, 40-in FFD, 12:1 grid
   C. 12.5 mAs, 70 kV, 40-in FFD, 16:1 grid
   D. 10 mAs, 70 kV, 50-in FFD, 5:1 grid

267. Which of the following radiographic techniques would produce a radiograph with the shortest scale of contrast?
   A. 200 mA, 0.25 sec, 90 kV, no grid, 3-in OFD
   B. 400 mA, 0.10 sec, 68 kV, 10:1 grid, 5-in OFD
   C. 300 mA, 0.50 sec, 82 kV, 8:1 grid, 2-in OFD
   D. 100 mA, 0.60 sec, 74 kV, 6:1 grid, 6-in OFD

268. In order to produce a 2× magnification for the cranium in the lateral position, if the FFD is 40 in, the OFD should be
   A. 10 in
   B. 20 in
   C. 25 in
   D. 30 in

269. Size distortion will increase when
   1. object-film distance is increased
   2. focus-film distance is decreased
   3. object is in poor alignment with focus and film
   A. 1 and 2 only
   B. 1 and 3 only
   C. 2 and 3 only
   D. 1, 2, and 3

270. In order to overcome magnification, when employing a 6-in OFD air gap for chest radiography, one should use an FFD of
   A. 36 in
   B. 48 in
   C. 72 in
   D. 120 in

271. The geometric unsharpness of margins with the radiographic image is referred to as the
1. umbra
2. penumbra
3. edge gradient

    A. 1 only
    B. 2 only
    C. 1 and 3 only
    D. 2 and 3 only

272. When a technologist is comparing two radiographs of the chest, one taken with a 72-in FFD and the other taken with a 50-in FFD (and a compensated technique), the radiograph with the 50-in FFD would exhibit
    A. increased distortion of the heart
    B. less autonomic motion
    C. greater definition
    D. increased quantum mottle

273. The **CORRECT** formula for calculating geometric unsharpness is UG equals
    A. $\dfrac{\text{Size of focal spot} \times \text{OFD}}{\text{FFD}}$
    B. $\text{OFD} \times \text{FFD}$
    C. Size of focal spot $\times$ FFD + OFD
    D. FFD $\times$ OFD $\times$ intensification factor

274. Which of the following is a method of reducing motion and decreasing the effects of fatty tissue?
    A. Use of cones
    B. Use of bucky device
    C. Compression device
    D. Increasing kilovoltage

275. Which of the following conditions is unrelated to a high incidence of penumbra?
    A. Short TFD
    B. Large effective focal spot
    C. Long OFD
    D. High kVp

276. Which of the following changes will affect radiographic contrast?
1. A change in grid ratio
2. A 15% change in kVp
3. A decrease in field size
   A. 1 and 2 only
   B. 1 and 3 only
   C. 2 and 3 only
   D. 1, 2, and 3

277. Which of the following changes would have a dramatic effect on radiographic contrast?
   A. Changing from 86 to 82 kVp
   B. Changing from a small to a large focal spot
   C. Changing from 100 to 125 mAs
   D. Changing from table-top to a 12:1 grid

278. Penumbra can be lessened by increasing the
   A. OFD
   B. SID
   C. mAs
   D. kVp

279. A supine chest taken at a 40-in SID will demonstrate
   A. maximum detail
   B. air and fluid levels
   C. a larger heart size
   D. true lung size

280. All other factors being compensated for, which of the following would produce the greatest radiographic definition if patient motion is a problem?
   A. 100 mA, 1/10 sec
   B. 200 mA, 1/20 sec
   C. 300 mA, 1/30 sec
   D. 400 mA, 1/40 sec

281. Which type of motion is usually present when a seriously injured patient is radiographed?
   A. Voluntary
   B. Involuntary
   C. Autonomic
   D. Physiological

282. Focal-film distance influences which of the following?
   1. Magnification
   2. Recorded detail
   3. Density
   A. 1 and 2 only
   B. 1 and 3 only
   C. 2 and 3 only
   D. 1, 2, and 3

283. Factors that govern the geometric sharpness include
   1. focal spot size
   2. object image receptor distance (OID)
   3. contrast
   A. 1 and 2 only
   B. 1 and 3 only
   C. 2 and 3 only
   D. 1, 2, and 3

284. Which of the following is unrelated to recorded detail?
   A. Immobilization of the body part
   B. Amount of thermionic emission
   C. Distance
   D. Focal spot size

285. Which of the following positions of the skull would produce a view of the frontal bone with the greatest amount of recorded detail?
   A. Caldwell
   B. Semiaxial AP
   C. Waters
   D. PA

286. Which of the following factors will directly influence recorded detail?
  1. Object-film distance
  2. Focus-film distance
  3. Focal spot size
  A. 1 and 2 only
  B. 1 and 3 only
  C. 2 and 3 only
  D. 1, 2, and 3

287. Listed below are four possible sets of technical factors to be used in a routine radiograph of a particular anatomic region. Select the set of factors that would most likely produce a radiograph with the **BEST** recorded detail.

	mAs	kVp	Part-film distance	Focal-film distance	Focal-spot size	Screen speed
A.	10	60	3 in	36 in	2.0 mm	High
B.	20	68	4 in	36 in	2.0 mm	Medium
C.	25	72	2 in	40 in	1.0 mm	Slow
D.	30	86	2 in	36 in	1.0 mm	Medium

288. Which of the following directly affects definition?
  1. Focal spot size
  2. mAs
  3. OFD
  A. 1 and 2 only
  B. 1 and 3 only
  C. 2 and 3 only
  D. 1, 2, and 3

289. Definition is impaired by
  1. increased OFD
  2. decreased FFD
  3. motion
  A. 1 and 2 only
  B. 1 and 3 only
  C. 2 and 3 only
  D. 1, 2, and 3

290. The smaller the effective focal spot, the
   A. greater the loss in definition
   B. greater the tube capacity
   C. lower the kV
   D. sharper the radiographic image

291. Which of the following is a contributing factor in producing recorded detail?
   A. Grid ratio
   B. Screen speed
   C. kVp
   D. mAs

292. Definition is directly influenced by the
   A. wavelength used
   B. tissue opacity
   C. OFD
   D. mAs

293. Which of the following is unrelated to recorded detail?
   A. Immobilization of the body part
   B. Distance
   C. Amount of thermionic emission
   D. Speed of the screen

294. Definition as applied to radiography refers to
   A. sharpness or clarity of the image
   B. variability in densities
   C. range of densities in the image
   D. degree of latitude visible

295. Which of the following is the **BEST** reason for using the shortest exposure time in chest radiography?
   A. Improves contrast
   B. Minimizes material unsharpness
   C. Minimizes shape distortion
   D. Eliminates physiologic motion

296. Which of the following combinations results in the **BEST** definition?
  A. Slow-speed screens and a 1-mm focal spot
  B. Medium-speed screens and a 1.5-mm focal spot
  C. High-speed screens and a 1.8-mm focal spot
  D. Rare-earth screens and a 2.0-mm focal spot

297. Which of the following sets of factors will exhibit the **BEST** definition of the carpal bones?
  1. 400 mAs, 60 kV, high-speed screens, 10-in air gap
  2. 200 mAs, 70 kV, medium-speed screens, long OFD
  3. 100 mAs, 50 kV, nonscreen film, short OFD
  A. 1 only
  B. 2 only
  C. 3 only
  D. 1, 2, and 3

298. Which of the following is usually lost during a change of 100 mA at 1/2 sec to 200 mA at 1/4 sec?
  A. Radiographic contrast
  B. Overall density
  C. True image size
  D. Sharp definition

299. Which of the following techniques would produce the greatest definition for a lateral cervical spine?
  A. 200 mA, 1/10 sec, 90 kV, 8-in OFD, 40-in FFD, high-speed screens
  B. 300 mA, 1/20 sec, 80 kV, 6-in OFD, 36-in FFD, par-speed screens
  C. 400 mA, 1/60 sec, 75 kV, 4-in OFD, 72-in FFD, slow-speed screens
  D. 500 mA, 1/120 sec, 60 kV, 4-in OFD, 48-in FFD, high-speed screens

300. A radiograph showing a complete lack of penumbra would be called
  A. sharp in detail
  B. low in density
  C. distorted
  D. magnified

301. Which of the following techniques would exhibit the highest amount of recorded detail?
- **A.** 100 mA, 1/10 sec, 60 kV, 48-in SID, 8-in OFD
- **B.** 200 mA, 1/15 sec, 65 kV, 60-in SID, 6-in OFD
- **C.** 400 mA, 1/30 sec, 70 kV, 72-in SID, 4-in OFD
- **D.** 600 mA, 1/60 sec, 80 kV, 120-in SID, 2-in OFD

302. Which of the following sets of technical factors would exhibit the **GREATEST** definition?
- **A.** 25 mAs, 90 kV, 32-in SID, high-speed screens
- **B.** 20 mAs, 80 kV, 40-in SID, high-speed screens
- **C.** 15 mAs, 75 kV, 42-in SID, medium-speed screens
- **D.** 10 mAs, 65 kV, 48-in SID, slow-speed screens

303. Which of the following radiographic techniques would produce a radiograph with the greatest recorded detail?
- **A.** 100 mA, 0.03 sec, 70 kV, 1-mm focal spot, 40-in SID, 4-in OFD
- **B.** 200 mA, 0.05 sec, 65 kV, 1-mm focal spot, 60-in SID, 1-in OFD
- **C.** 300 mA, 0.25 sec, 60 kV, 2-mm focal spot, 50-in SID, 1-in OFD
- **D.** 300 mA, 0.40 sec, 55 kV, 2-mm focal spot, 35-in SID, 3-in OFD

304. Which of the following radiographic techniques would exhibit the greatest density?
- **A.** 75 mA, 1 sec, 80 kV, 6:1 grid
- **B.** 50 mA, 1.5 sec, 60 kV, 10:1 grid
- **C.** 200 mA, 0.25 sec, 70 kV, 8:1 grid
- **D.** 300 mA, 0.33 sec, 65 kV, 12:1 grid

305. 300 mAs is obtained by selecting
  1. 450 mA at 0.66 sec
  2. 1200 mA at 0.25 sec
  3. 600 mA at 0.50 sec
- **A.** 1 only
- **B.** 1 and 2 only
- **C.** 2 and 3 only
- **D.** 1, 2, and 3

306. Which statement properly relates to the three techniques regarding density?

  1. 200 mA, 60 kV, high-speed screen, 36-in FFD
  2. 350 mA, 70 kV, medium-speed screen, 48-in FFD
  3. 800 mA, 80 kV, slow-speed screen, 72-in FFD

  A. Choice 2 exhibits the greatest density
  B. All three techniques are basically equal
  C. Choice 1 exhibits the greatest density
  D. Choice 3 exhibits the greatest density

307. If a lateral skull were radiographed at 200 mA, 1/5 sec, 70 kV, 40-in FFD and the film were light, which of the following adjustments would produce a noticeable change?

  A. 100 mA, 1/2 sec, 70 kV
  B. 200 mA, 3/20 sec, 72 kV
  C. 400 mA, 1/10 sec, 73 kV
  D. 300 mA, 1/5 sec, 70 kV

308. A technique of 200 mA, 1/4 sec has been used to produce a film of satisfactory density. If the mA were changed to 500, the time needed to obtain the same mAs, all other factors remaining constant, would be

  A. 3/20 sec
  B. 2/10 sec
  C. 1/15 sec
  D. 1/10 sec

309. Which of the following mA selections is needed to produce radiographs with equal density when the original technique of 300 mA, 1/40 sec, high-speed screen, 16:1 grid is changed to 1/20 sec, medium-speed screen, 8:1 grid?

  A. 100 mA
  B. 200 mA
  C. 400 mA
  D. 600 mA

310. Which of the following sets of technical factors would produce a radiograph with the greatest density?
  A. 1000 mA, 1/120 sec, 75 kV, 48-in SID, 5:1 grid
  B. 700 mA, 1/20 sec, 72 kV, 40-in SID, 6:1 grid
  C. 600 mA, 1/40 sec, 76 kV, 54-in SID, 10:1 grid
  D. 300 mA, 1/10 sec, 74 kV, 52-in SID, 12:1 grid

311. A change of 100 mA to 300 mA will
  1. cause more thermionic emission to occur
  2. alter the penetrating ability
  3. increase the number of photons produced
  A. 1 and 2 only
  B. 1 and 3 only
  C. 2 and 3 only
  D. 1, 2, and 3

312. A skull is normally radiographed using 300 mA, 1/10 second, and 70 kVp. What new mAs would be used to produce a similar radiograph at 91 kVp?
  A. 5.0 mAs
  B. 7.5 mAs
  C. 10.0 mAs
  D. 15.0 mAs

313. A technique of 200 mA, 1/2 sec, 70 kV, 40-in FFD is changed to 1200 mA at 60 kV and 40-in FFD to improve contrast and eliminate motion. What new time is also needed to maintain the original density?
  A. 1/3 sec
  B. 1/4 sec
  C. 1/5 sec
  D. 1/6 sec

314. Which of the following combinations of mAs would be ideal for an uncooperative or irrational patient requiring a KUB?
  A. 100 mA, 1.0 sec
  B. 200 mA, 0.5 sec
  C. 500 mA, 0.20 sec
  D. 1000 mA, 0.01 sec

315. Which of the following radiographic techniques would produce the greatest quantity of photons?
- **A.** 200 mA, 0.75 sec
- **B.** 400 mA, 0.25 sec
- **C.** 500 mA, 0.10 sec
- **D.** 600 mA, 0.40 sec

316. If an original mA of 300 and an exposure time of 1/12 of a second were used, and you changed the mA to 400, what new exposure time would be needed in order to maintain the original density?
- **A.** 1/10 sec
- **B.** 1/14 sec
- **C.** 1/16 sec
- **D.** 1/20 sec

317. If the standard is 200 mA, 1/10 sec, 60 kV, medium-speed screens, the adjustment should be 200 mA, 60 kV, high-speed screens, at how many seconds?
- **A.** 1/40 sec
- **B.** 1/20 sec
- **C.** 1/10 sec
- **D.** 1/5 sec

318. An initial radiograph was taken applying the following factors: 200 mAs, 3/10 seconds, 70 kV, 40-in FFD. Another radiograph is required, but the circumstances are such that the only available FFD is 30 in. In order to maintain radiographic density, the corrected mAs would be approximately
- **A.** 15 mAs
- **B.** 20 mAs
- **C.** 28 mAs
- **D.** 34 mAs

319. A technique for a 10-cm knee table top is 100 mA, 1/30 sec, 55 kV. The radiologist requests that an additional film be taken utilizing a 12:1 ratio grid. Which of the following techniques would represent the proper conversion from the original technique?
- **A.** 200 mA, 1/15 sec, 70 kV
- **B.** 100 mA, 1/6 sec, 55 kV
- **C.** 300 mA, 1/30 sec, 60 kV
- **D.** 50 mA, 1/20 sec, 45 kV

320. Which combinations of exposure factors will give the highest radiographic density?
   A. 50 mA, 1.5 sec, 72 kV, 12:1 grid
   B. 50 mA, 1/2 sec, 80 kV, 6:1 grid
   C. 150 mA, 1/2 sec, 70 kV, 16:1 grid
   D. 200 mA, 3/8 sec, 76 kV, 6:1 grid

321. If a 7-cm ankle can be satisfactorily radiographed at 100 mA, 1/10 sec, 60 kV, 40-in FFD without a grid, which of the following techniques could be used for a 12-cm knee to maintain the same density?
   1. 20 mAs, 60 kV, no grid
   2. 40 mAs, 70 kV, no grid
   3. 50 mAs, 60 kV, 10:1 grid
   A. 1 only
   B. 2 only
   C. 1 and 3 only
   D. 1, 2, and 3

322. A radiograph is produced with optimum density using 100 mAs at 80 kVp. Which of the following exposure factors will produce a radiograph with similar density, but increased contrast?
   A. 200 mAs at 68 kVp
   B. 200 mAs at 74 kVp
   C. 300 mAs at 86 kVp
   D. 450 mAs at 92 kVp

323. Which of the following radiographic techniques would have the highest incidence of scatter radiation?
   A. 100 mA, 1/15 sec, 75 kVp
   B. 200 mA, 1/30 sec, 80 kVp
   C. 300 mA, 1/60 sec, 90 kVp
   D. 400 mA, 1/120 sec, 100 kVp

324. If the milliampere selector were set at 1000 mA, what exposure time would be required to produce 80 mAs?
   A. 0.008 sec
   B. 0.08 sec
   C. 0.80 sec
   D. 8.0 sec

325. Which of the following exposure times represents 50 msec?
  1. 0.05 sec
  2. 1/20 sec
  3. 10 mA at 5 sec
  A. 1 only
  B. 1 and 2 only
  C. 2 and 3 only
  D. 1, 2, and 3

326. A technique of 100 mA, 1/2 sec at 80 kV should be converted to 50 mA, 2 sec at how many kV to maintain the same density?
  A. 60 kV
  B. 70 kV
  C. 92 kV
  D. 105 kV

327. An x-ray machine that is properly calibrated will guarantee a duplication of radiographic density with a technique of 100 mA, 1/2 sec, and a technique of
  A. 400 mA, 1/16 sec
  B. 200 mA, 1/4 sec
  C. 50 mA, 1/4 sec
  D. 25 mA, 1 sec

328. If a knee was radiographed at 100 mA, 1/20 sec, 64 kV, TT, and we converted to a 10:1 grid to improve contrast, the properly adjusted technique would be
  A. 100 mA, 1/5 sec, 64 kV
  B. 200 mA, 1/8 sec, 64 kV
  C. 100 mA, 1 sec, 64 kV
  D. 100 mA, 1/4 sec, 64 kV

329. Which technique would produce a film with the **MOST** density?
  A. 100 mA, 1/2 sec, 72 kV, high-speed screens
  B. 200 mA, 1/4 sec, 76 kV, par-speed screens
  C. 400 mA, 1/3 sec, 82 kV, high-speed screens
  D. 600 mA, 1/6 sec, 84 kV, slow-speed screens

330. Which technique would produce the **MOST** density?
   A. 1000 mA, 0.040 sec
   B. 700 mA, 0.025 sec
   C. 400 mA, 0.15 sec
   D. 300 mA, 0.07 sec

331. At which of the following exposure times does 200 mA at 0.5 sec convert to an equivalent mAs of 500 mA?
   A. 0.1 sec
   B. 0.2 sec
   C. 0.4 sec
   D. 1.0 sec

332. A radiograph is taken of the lumbar spine with a technique of 100 mA, 1 sec at 80 kV. If the technique were adjusted to 100 mA, 1/2 sec at 90 kV, which of the following would be **TRUE**?
   A. The overall density would decrease
   B. There would be a decrease of 3,500 HU
   C. There would be an increase of 4,500 HU
   D. The HU would increase from 8,000 to 16,000

333. Which of the following techniques would produce the **LEAST** density?
   A. 200 mA, 1/2 sec, 78 kV, 40-in SID
   B. 150 mA, 1/6 sec, 88 kV, 50-in SID
   C. 50 mA, 1 sec, 72 kV, 40-in SID
   D. 200 mA, 1/8 sec, 75 kV, 60-in SID

334. Which of the following radiographic techniques would exhibit the greatest density?
   A. 150 mA, 1/5 sec, 60 kV, medium screen, 36-in FFD
   B. 400 mA, 1/20 sec, 70 kV, high screen, 36-in FFD
   C. 100 mA, 2/5 sec, 50 kV, high screen, 42-in FFD
   D. 300 mA, 1/10 sec, 60 kV, medium screen, 40-in FFD

335. Starting with the technique listed below, which of the following changes would **NOT** double the radiographic density? 200 mA, 1 sec, 60 kV, par-speed screens, 40-in FFD, 1-mm focal spot
   A. Increase the kV to 70
   B. Change to high-speed screens
   C. Increase the focal spot size to 2 mm
   D. Adjust the mAs to 400

336. Which of the following exposure times combined with 300 mA will yield 30 mAs?
   1. 100 msec
   2. 1/10 sec
   3. 0.1 sec
   A. 1 only
   B. 1 and 2 only
   C. 2 and 3 only
   D. 1, 2, and 3

337. If the mA was set at 300 and the mAs produced was 15, the exposure time would be
   A. 0.005 sec
   B. 0.05 sec
   C. 0.5 sec
   D. 5.0 sec

338. Collimation from a 14-in × 17-in field to an 8-in × 10-in field with all other factors remaining the same will result in a radiograph that exhibits
   A. increased contrast and decreased density
   B. decreased contrast and increased density
   C. increased contrast and increased density
   D. decreased contrast and decrease in image size

339. Which of the following changes would be the minimum required in order to visibly see a difference in film density?
   A. Change the original mAs by 30%
   B. Change the original mAs by 60%
   C. Change the kVp by 30%
   D. Change the kVp by 60%

340. Which of the following does **NOT** roughly double image density?
  A. 40- to 30-in SID
  B. 50 to 58 kVp
  C. 12:1 to 6:1 grid ratio
  D. 0.6- to 1.2-mm focal spot

341. A technique of 200 mA at 0.10 sec, and 70 kVp can be properly converted to maintain the original density to
  A. 200 mA at 0.50 sec, 80 kVp
  B. 400 mA at 0.05 sec, 70 kVp
  C. 600 mA at 0.125 sec, 60 kVp
  D. 800 mA at 0.025 sec, 90 kVp

342. Which of the following conversions from 200 mA, 1/2 sec, 65 kVp would demonstrate a visible change in density?
  A. 200 mA, 4/5 sec, 68 kVp
  B. 300 mA, 1/3 sec, 66 kVp
  C. 300 mA, 1/4 sec, 67 kVp
  D. 400 mA, 1/5 sec, 64 kVp

343. When a table-top knee radiograph demonstrates motion, the technique of 200 mA, 1/10 at 64 kVp can be properly converted to
  A. 200 mA, 1/20 sec, 54 kVp
  B. 400 mA, 1/40 sec, 64 kVp
  C. 800 mA, 1/80 sec, 73 kVp
  D. 1200 mA, 1/30 sec, 80 kVp

344. After ensuring patient understanding and cooperation, what is the **CHIEF** method of reducing the effect of physiologic motion on the film?
  A. Reduction of exposure time
  B. Immobilization of the part
  C. Decreasing focal spot size
  D. Decreasing screen speed

345. Which combination of 30 mAs is ideal for an uncooperative patient?
   A. 200 mA at 0.15 sec
   B. 300 mA at 1/10 sec
   C. 500 mA at 0.06 sec
   D. 600 mA at 1/20 sec

346. In order to maintain the sharpest definition on a radiograph it would be **BEST** to change a technique of 100 mA, 1/2 sec to
   A. 200 mA, 1/4 sec
   B. leave mA at 100, increase kV approximately 30
   C. the highest mA value and fastest exposure time, but maintaining 50 mÁs
   D. the fastest exposure time possible and highest mA available

347. A femoral arteriogram exposure calls for a radiographic technique of 70 mAs at 80 kV. If the generator has a capacity of 1000 mA, the fastest possible exposure time in seconds would be
   A. 0.007
   B. 0.07
   C. 0.7
   D. 7.0

348. If the kilovoltage were at 46, how much of a minimum change would have to occur in order to produce a noticeable increase in density, such as a doubling in density?
   A. 2 kV
   B. 7 kV
   C. 15 kV
   D. 20 to 25 kV

349. To convert, maintaining the same density, the technique of nongrid, 60 mAs, 70 kV, 80-in FFD to 6:1 grid, 22.5 mAs, 40-in FFD, how many kV would be required?
   A. 60 kV
   B. 76 kV
   C. 80 kV
   D. 92 kV

350. A radiograph that exhibits a long-scale of contrast is one in which there are
   A. many shades of gray with minimal difference in density between each shade
   B. few shades of gray with great difference in density between each shade
   C. many shades of gray with great difference in density between each shade
   D. few shades of gray with minimal difference in density between each shade

351. When the kV is **INCREASED,** the x-ray tube produces a beam that is of
   A. lower frequency and greater quantity
   B. longer wavelengths and lower frequency
   C. higher frequency and shorter wavelengths
   D. lesser quality and greater homogeneity

352. The air gap technique improves
   A. magnification and distortion
   B. radiography contrast
   C. film density
   D. edge gradient

353. Which of the following radiographic techniques would produce the greatest density and longest scale of contrast?
   A. 50 mA, 0.10 sec, 64 kV, 10:1 grid
   B. 100 mA, 0.15 sec, 66 kV, 6:1 grid
   C. 150 mA, 0.25 sec, 68 kV, no grid
   D. 200 mA, 0.30 sec, 72 kV, 8:1 grid

354. Which of the following factors does **NOT** affect subject contrast?
   A. kVp
   B. mA
   C. Object shape and size
   D. Tissue density

355. If a radiographic technique of 200 mA, 0.5 sec, at 120 kVp is used for an abdomen measuring 34 cm, which of the following would be essential in order to maintain radiographic contrast?
  A. Using the smallest focal spot
  B. Using a high-ratio grid
  C. Using a field size larger than 14 in × 17 in
  D. Removing all filtration

356. If the milliamperage were reduced from 200 mA to 100 mA, the kilovoltage could be increased to maintain the same density from 100 kV to
  A. 108 kV
  B. 110 kV
  C. 115 kV
  D. 125 kV

357. The number of structural lines actually recorded within a radiographic image is referred to as image
  A. resolution
  B. contrast
  C. visibility
  D. quality

358. The density on a radiograph can be doubled by
  A. cutting the distance in half
  B. going down a step in exposure time
  C. increasing the kVp by 15%
  D. increasing the mAs by 30%

359. An adjustment in the kilovoltage from 60 to 80 will produce
  1. an increase in latitude
  2. less patient absorption
  3. shorter wavelengths
  A. 1 and 2 only
  B. 1 and 3 only
  C. 2 and 3 only
  D. 1, 2, and 3

360. Which of the following anatomic structures should exhibit the highest subject contrast?
A. Lung
B. Bladder
C. Heart
D. Femur

361. When changing from a medium-speed screen to a high-speed screen, there will be a decrease in the necessary amount of exposure and increased
A. latitude
B. resolution
C. contrast
D. detail

362. The original exposure factors are 200 mA, 86 kV, and 1/2 sec. What would the new exposure time have to be if the kV were reduced to 80?
A. 1/6 sec
B. 1/4 sec
C. 2/5 sec
D. 3/4 sec

363. The **GREATEST** amount of geometric unsharpness is usually attributed to the factor of
A. size of focus
B. FFD
C. screen speed
D. OFD

364. A lateral skull radiograph on a child taken at 200 mA, 1/5 sec, 85 kVp shows unacceptable amounts of scatter radiation. A logical change would be to
A. increase grid ratio
B. reduce kVp
C. utilize the air gap principle
D. use higher-speed screens

365. Size distortion will **INCREASE** when
1. OFD is increased
2. FFD is decreased
3. the object is in poor alignment with focus and film
- **A.** 1 and 2 only
- **B.** 1 and 3 only
- **C.** 2 and 3 only
- **D.** 1, 2, and 3

366. An exposure taken at 20 mAs, 80 kV, at 72 in demonstrates a satisfactory radiograph. What new mAs would be needed if the kilovoltage remained at 80, but the FFD were reduced to 56 in?
- **A.** 8 mAs
- **B.** 12 mAs
- **C.** 40 mAs
- **D.** 80 mAs

367. To compensate for an **INCREASE** in distance from 24 to 48 in, the technologist could
1. increase the kV approximately 20%
2. multiply the mAs by four
3. change from par- to high-speed screens and double the mAs
- **A.** 1 and 2 only
- **B.** 1 and 3 only
- **C.** 2 and 3 only
- **D.** 1, 2, and 3

368. Increasing geometric unsharpness principally affects
- **A.** sensitivity
- **B.** resolution
- **C.** contrast
- **D.** density

369. If a radiographic technique of 300 mA, 1/5 sec, 70 kV produces 80 mR at 40 in, what would a technique of 400 mA, 1/3 sec, 70 kV produce at 40 in?
   A. 90 mR
   B. 120 mR
   C. 160 mR
   D. 360 mR

370. If the original technique for a radiograph which calls for a 40-in TFD and 0.5 seconds is changed to a 20-in TFD and the addition of an 8:1 grid, what would the new exposure time have to be in order to maintain the same density?
   A. 0.10 sec
   B. 0.25 sec
   C. 1.0 sec
   D. No change

371. A chest radiograph is exposed at 300 mA, 1 sec, 80 kV, at 200 cm. In order to maintain density, what new exposure time is required at 100 cm?
   A. 0.025 sec
   B. 0.05 sec
   C. 0.2 sec
   D. 0.4 sec

372. If 700 mA at 2/10 sec, 80-in FFD gives a sufficient density, what new time is needed when using 700 mA at 40-in FFD to give the same density?
   A. 4/5 sec
   B. 1/10 sec
   C. 1/20 sec
   D. 1/40 sec

373. When 100 mAs is produced at an SID of 40 in, how much mAs is needed at a 30-in SID in order to maintain original density?
   A. 56.25 mAs
   B. 59.25 mAs
   C. 62.50 mAs
   D. 66.25 mAs

374. Which of the following conversions is **INCORRECT** when converting a table-top knee technique of 100 mA, 1/20 sec, 64 kV, and 40-in FFD to a bucky?
  A. 200 mA, 1/10 sec, 64 kV, 40-in FFD, 8:1 grid
  B. 100 mA, 1/25 sec, 64 kV, 40-in FFD, 10:1 grid
  C. 500 mA, 1/20 sec, 64 kV, 40-in FFD, 12:1 grid
  D. 100 mA, 3/10 sec, 64 kV, 40-in FFD, 16:1 grid

375. All other factors being unchanged, if a technique of 75 mAs with a 5:1 grid were changed to use an 8:1 grid, what would the new mAs have to be?
  A. 37.5 mAs
  B. 112 mAs
  C. 150 mAs
  D. 300 mAs

376. To maintain the same density, what would the new exposure time have to be if a technique of 200 mA at 1/5 sec, nongrid were changed to include the use of a 12:1 grid?
  A. 1/25 sec
  B. 1/10 sec
  C. 4/5 sec
  D. 1 sec

377. If a technique of 120 mAs with a 10:1 grid is changed to use a 6:1 grid, what would the new mAs have to be?
  A. 60 mAs
  B. 72 mAs
  C. 80 mAs
  D. 240 mAs

378. A technique of 100 mAs at 90 kVp, 8:1 grid can be properly converted to a 5:1 grid, 80 kVp at
  A. 25 mAs
  B. 50 mAs
  C. 100 mAs
  D. 200 mAs

379. A technique of 100 mAs at 90 kVp with a 12:1 grid could be properly converted to a 6:1 grid at 76 kV at
    A. 50 mAs
    B. 80 mAs
    C. 100 mAs
    D. 120 mAs

380. A technique of 80 mAs, 75 kVp nongrid could be properly converted to a 6:1 grid, 86 kVp at
    A. 100 mAs
    B. 120 mAs
    C. 140 mAs
    D. 160 mAs

381. If a chest is radiographed at 200 mA, 0.03 sec, medium-speed screens, and exhibits an appropriate density, what new exposure time would maintain the original density if high-speed screens are used?
    A. 0.003 sec
    B. 0.015 sec
    C. 0.06 sec
    D. 0.30 sec

382. Quantum mottle would **MOST** likely occur when using
    A. rare-earth screens
    B. par-speed screens
    C. ultra-detail screens
    D. nonscreen film holders

383. When a portion of the radiographic image appears blurred, it is due to
    A. inadequate collimation
    B. poor film screen contact
    C. excessive kilovoltage
    D. slow grid movement

384. If an AP elbow radiographed at 100 mA, 0.03 sec, 60 kVp, par-speed needs to be repeated because of motion, the radiographer would use a high-speed screen at
- A. 50 mA, 0.03 sec, 68 kVp
- B. 100 mA, 0.03 sec, 68 kVp
- C. 100 mA, 0.015 sec, 60 kVp
- D. 200 mA, 0.03 sec, 60 kVp

385. The manifest image is composed of
- A. silver halide
- B. calcium tungstate
- C. strontium sulfate
- D. metallic silver crystals

386. The average base plus fog level on radiographic film will produce densitometer readings of about
- A. 0 to 0.5
- B. 0.05 to 0.15
- C. 0.15 to 0.50
- D. 0.50 to 1.0

387. When a 6-in air gap is used in chest radiography, which of the following statements would be **TRUE**?
- A. a 72-in FFD is needed for true heart and lung size
- B. the kilovoltage should be raised to 120
- C. a low-ratio grid is required
- D. soft pulmonary infiltrates and small densities are well-demonstrated

388. Which of the following has an effect on the production of secondary and scattered radiations?
- 1. Thickness of the part being x-rayed
- 2. Density of the tissue being x-rayed
- 3. Kilovoltage
- A. 1 and 2 only
- B. 1 and 3 only
- C. 2 and 3 only
- D. 1, 2, and 3

389. The invisible image that is produced in the film emulsion by exposure to light or x-rays is called the
   A. latent image
   B. manifest image
   C. radiologic image
   D. photographic image

390. Which of the following devices will reduce the amount of scattered radiation reaching the film?
   1. Beam restrictors
   2. Filters
   3. Grids
   A. 1 and 2 only
   B. 1 and 3 only
   C. 2 and 3 only
   D. 1, 2, and 3

391. Grid frequency is defined as the
   A. ratio of lead strip height to lead strip thickness
   B. ratio of lead strip height to interspace thickness
   C. speed of the reciprocating grid
   D. number of lead strips per inch

392. Which of the following body parts is usually radiographed table top?
   A. AP, 15-cm knee
   B. Internal rotation, 16-cm shoulder
   C. Lateral, 18-cm femur
   D. Postreduction, 8-cm lateral elbow

393. Close collimation will help control
   A. the use of large focal spots
   B. a high percentage of distortion
   C. the use of grids
   D. radiographic fog

394. Which of the following devices are employed to reduce patient exposure to x-rays?
    1. Grids
    2. Collimators
    3. Filters
    A. 1 and 2 only
    B. 1 and 3 only
    C. 2 and 3 only
    D. 1, 2, and 3

395. A 16:1 grid, compared to an 8:1 grid, will
    A. have a longer scale of contrast
    B. absorb more secondary radiation
    C. absorb more soft rays
    D. move faster in the bucky

396. Which of the following has a direct effect on the efficiency of a bucky grid in removing scattered radiation?
    A. Screen speed
    B. Field size
    C. Composition of table top
    D. Grid ratio

397. When radiographing the abdomen, which of the following would **DECREASE** the production of scatter radiation?
    A. Increased kilovoltage
    B. Use of high-speed screens
    C. Proper collimation
    D. Use of a small focal spot

398. A grid that has lead strips 0.25 mm apart and 4 mm high will have a ratio of
    A. 6:1
    B. 8:1
    C. 10:1
    D. 16:1

399. Which type of grid has lead lines running only in one direction?
  A. Cross-hatched
  B. Linear
  C. Rhombic
  D. Focus

400. Grid ratio is expressed by which of the following formulas?
  A. $R = D \times H$
  B. $R = \dfrac{D}{H}$
  C. $R = \dfrac{I}{D + H}$
  D. $R = \dfrac{H}{D}$

401. The use of a grid will protect the
  A. patient from primary radiation
  B. film from scattered radiation
  C. patient from scattered radiation
  D. film from primary radiation

402. Barium sulphate on the film surface of a cassette would cause an artifact that would appear as a
  A. low-contrast mark
  B. high-definition spot
  C. high-density mark
  D. low-density spot

403. The anode heel effect is an important consideration when taking radiographs of the
  A. skull
  B. wrist
  C. ankle
  D. femur

404. The heel effect becomes more pronounced as the
1. anode angle decreases
2. film size increases
3. FFD decreases
   A. 1 only
   B. 1 and 2 only
   C. 2 and 3 only
   D. 1, 2, and 3

405. Which of the following are affected by filtration of the x-ray beam?
1. Exposure rate
2. Half-value layer
3. Recorded definition
   A. 1 and 2 only
   B. 1 and 3 only
   C. 2 and 3 only
   D. 1, 2, and 3

406. Geometric unsharpness is **NOT** influenced by
   A. size of focal spot
   B. focal-film distance (SID)
   C. object-film distance
   D. thickness of the part examined

407. When the x-ray beam passes through a filter, which of the following occurs?
1. Greater penetration of beam
2. Improved attenuation of long-wave photons
3. Increased beam quality
   A. 1 only
   B. 1 and 2 only
   C. 2 and 3 only
   D. 1, 2, and 3

408. An adjustment in the kilovoltage from 60 to 80 will produce
    1. an increase in latitude
    2. less patient absorption
    3. shorter wavelength radiation
  A. 1 and 2 only
  B. 1 and 3 only
  C. 2 and 3 only
  D. 1, 2, and 3

409. In order to prevent pressure marks, x-ray film should be stored
  A. on the floor of the darkroom
  B. on end
  C. in the diagnostic room
  D. in stacks

410. The silver halide latent image is produced by
  A. sodium sulfite
  B. acetic acid
  C. x-rays, light, or other forms of radiation
  D. developing agents

411. The tinting used in some radiographic intensifying screens keeps the visible light from spreading, and also
  A. decreases recorded detail and decreases screen speed
  B. decreases recorded detail and increases screen speed
  C. increases recorded detail and decreases screen speed
  D. increases recorded detail and increases screen speed

412. Much of the contrast on radiographic films in diagnostic radiography is due to
  A. the Compton effect
  B. coherent scattering
  C. pair production
  D. the photoelectric effect

413. The radiographic film base appears blue
  A. because of added hardeners
  B. so that viewing the image will be more pleasant
  C. to match the light emitted by the intensifying screens
  D. because of the silver halide crystals

414. The visible image is composed of
  A. sodium carbonate crystals
  B. potassium bromide crystals
  C. metallic silver grains
  D. hydroquinone and elon

415. Phototimer cassettes differ from conventional cassettes in that
  A. the front is not radiolucent
  B. phototimer cassettes have radiolucent backs
  C. they do not have hinges
  D. they cannot be made of bakelite

416. The layer of the intensifying screen closest to the film is the
  A. base
  B. protective coating
  C. phosphor layer
  D. reflective layer

417. Gadolinium and lanthanum compounds are
  A. special reducing agents found in the developer
  B. iodinated radiographic contrast agents
  C. high-speed rare-earth phosphors
  D. gallbladder evacuants

418. Assuring good film-screen contact also assures reduced
  A. contrast levels
  B. geometric unsharpness
  C. absorption unsharpness
  D. material unsharpness

419. Poor film screen contact results in
A. additional density
B. decreased definition
C. varied contrast levels
D. increased penumbra

420. The base layer in the intensifying screen can be made of
A. titanium dioxide
B. polyester
C. zinc sulfide
D. calcium tungstate

421. The intensification factor of screens refers to their
A. speed
B. resolution
C. lag
D. density

422. Phosphorescence is the name given to
A. a drop in voltage during exposure
B. continued fluoroscence of screen after x-ray is terminated
C. the period of time elapsed after the circuit is closed and x-ray is produced
D. a delay in grid movement

423. The emulsion of x-ray film consists of a mixture of homogeneous
   1. gelatin
   2. cellulose nitrate
   3. silver halide crystals
A. 1 only
B. 1 and 2 only
C. 1 and 3 only
D. 1, 2, and 3

424. The condition of osteolysis would require
　　1. the use of a large focal spot
　　2. a decrease in exposure factors
　　3. the utilization of a high-ratio grid
　A. 1 only
　B. 2 only
　C. 1 and 2 only
　D. 1, 2, and 3

425. Which of the following is(are) considered to be radiotransparent?
　　1. Iodinated compounds
　　2. Carbon dioxide
　　3. Air
　A. 1 only
　B. 2 only
　C. 2 and 3 only
　D. 1, 2, and 3

426. Which of the following anatomical parts would attenuate the **MOST** radiation?
　A. Ilium
　B. Pleura
　C. Psoas muscle
　D. Liver

427. If a forearm is satisfactorily radiographed at 100 mA, 1/20 sec, and 60 kV, what is the appropriate postreduction technique?
　A. 5 mAs, 54 kV
　B. 10 mAs, 66 kV
　C. 20 mAs, 80 kV
　D. 40 mAs, 62 kV

428. The logical technique change for a patient with tachypnea who requires a chest radiograph would be to
　A. decrease the penetration
　B. decrease the beam's quantity
　C. limit the field of exposure
　D. change to high-speed screens and decrease exposure time

429. A technique of 100 mA, 1/20 sec at 60 kV was used to expose a fractured forearm adequately. What technique would be **BEST** to use after a cast has been applied?

    A. 100 mA, 1/20 sec, 75 kV (+15% kV)
    B. 400 mA, 1/20 sec, 60 kV (8 × mAs)
    C. 200 mA, 1/20 sec, 66 kV (2 × mAs + 10% kVp)
    D. 100 mA, 1/10 sec, 80 kVp (2 × mAs + 20% kVp)

430. Which of the following conditions requires a **DECREASE** in the normal exposure factors to penetrate the part properly?

    A. Pneumoconiosis
    B. Advanced carcinoma
    C. Atelectasis
    D. Atrophy

431. A **DECREASE** in kilovoltage is required for

    A. osteomalacia
    B. pleural effusion
    C. sclerosis
    D. osteopetrosis

432. Which of the following qualities of a radiographic film will be **MOST** improved by the use of a compression band, applied to areas with excessive amounts of soft tissue?

    A. Density
    B. Contrast
    C. Detail
    D. Magnification

433. In which of the following pathological conditions should the technologist **DECREASE** normal exposure factors?

    A. Pulmonary edema
    B. Ascites
    C. Pleural effusion
    D. Emphysema

434. The presence of ascites will result in an **INCREASE** of
  A. density
  B. scattered radiation
  C. distortion
  D. contrast

435. Voluntary motion caused by mental illness or age can be controlled only by
  A. giving clear instructions
  B. speed of exposure
  C. supporting immobilization
  D. providing comfort for the patient

436. Which statement is **INCORRECT** regarding penetrability of x-rays to pathology?
  A. Neuroblastoma requires a reduction in factors
  B. Multiple myeloma requires additional factors
  C. Pneumothorax requires a reduction in factors
  D. Edema requires additional factors

437. Which of the following conditions requires additional radiographic technique to penetrate?
  A. Gout
  B. Carcinoma
  C. Fibrosarcoma
  D. Empyema

438. Which of the following conditions requires a reduction in technical factors?
  A. Hydropneumothorax
  B. Active tuberculosis
  C. Aortic aneurysm
  D. Acute kyphosis

439. Which of the following diseases require a **DECREASE** in the penetrating ability of x-radiation?
    1. Emphysema
    2. Osteoporosis
    3. Pleural effusion
  A. 1 and 2 only
  B. 1 and 3 only
  C. 2 and 3 only
  D. 1, 2, and 3

440. Two developing agents are combined to produce
  A. a very short contrast scale
  B. good detail and moderate-to-high contrast
  C. high density in the radiograph
  D. protection of the image

441. The component of the developing solution that helps keep unexposed silver crystals from the reducing agent is
  A. hydroquinon
  B. phenidone
  C. sodium carbonate
  D. potassium bromide

442. The basic constituents in a developer are
  A. sulfuric acid, sodium carbonate, and potassium
  B. accelerator, preservative, and developing agents
  C. sodium chloride, sodium hydroxide, and restrainers
  D. chrome alum, hyposulfite, and bromine

443. The presence of the restrainer inhibits
  A. oxidation
  B. evaporation
  C. overdevelopment
  D. fogging

444. The transport system of an automatic film processor
1. moves the film through the processor at a controlled speed
2. provides uniform agitation of solutions to the surface of the film
3. provides squeegee action to remove excess solution from the surface of the film
   A. 1 and 2 only
   B. 1 and 3 only
   C. 2 and 3 only
   D. 1, 2, and 3

445. Conversion of the latent image to a metallic silver image is accomplished by
A. washing and drying
B. ionization
C. development and fixation
D. tanning

446. The hardener in the fixing solution is
A. acetic acid
B. sodium carbonate
C. chrome alum
D. potassium hydroxide

447. In the automatic processor located between the fixing tank and wash tank is the
A. transportation rack
B. entrance roller
C. drying chamber
D. crossover rack

448. In order to provide **INCREASED** concentration of solutions in an automatic processor, the chemical used is
A. glutaraldehyde
B. potassium bromide
C. hydroquinone
D. phenidone

449. The developing time for screen-type film at 72° should be
   A. 3 min
   B. 4 min
   C. 5 min
   D. 6 min

450. The essential ingredients of the fixer are
   A. preservative, reducer, hardener, and acid
   B. acid, hardener, hypo, and preservative
   C. tanning agent, accelerator, reducer, and preservative
   D. alkali, preservative, reducer, and restrainer

Explanatory Answers

251. B. The useful diagnostic range of radiographic density lies between 0.4 to 2.75, as read on the densitometer. (Ref. 11, p. 119)

252. B. Examples of the body's naturally occurring densities, from the least to the most dense, are: gas, fat, cartilage, hollow organs (empty), muscle, solid organs, hollow organs (filled), and bone. (Ref. 11, p. 115)

253. B. As the OFD increases, scattered radiation is absorbed in an air gap, which eliminates use of a grid for chest radiography. (Ref. 11, p. 126)

254. B. Hollow organs, such as those in the gastrointestinal tract that are induced with contrast media, require additional beam quality because of their lack of adequate subject contrast in their natural state. (Ref. 11, p. 116)

255. D. A change in table-top exposure to a 12:1 grid, with a 5× increase in mAs to maintain density, would demonstrate a higher contrast. (Ref. 11, p. 144)

256. A. Long wavelengths relate to low kV ranges which produce a short-scale contrast in the image. (Ref. 11, p. 117)

257. A. Focal spot size does not affect radiographic contrast. Grid ratio and OFD (air gap) will affect the scale of contrast. (Ref. 11, p. 145)

258. C. Scattered radiation that would normally fog the film is absorbed by the air gap principle. (Ref. 11, p. 127)

259. B. By increasing the kVp above that needed to penetrate the tissue, the scale of contrast in the image is extended. (Ref. 11, p. 122)

260. B. Low contrast or long-scale contrast is an extension of the scale of contrast in the image consisting of many similar densities. (Ref. 11, p. 122)

261. B.   High kV produces a long scale of contrast in the image. (Ref. 11, p. 117)

262. B.   Short-scale contrast equals low kilovoltage and high grid ratio. Focal spot size has no effect. (Ref. 11, p. 144)

263. B.   Short-scale contrast equals high grid ratio, low kilovoltage, small field size, and high-speed screens. (Ref. 11, p. 145)

264. B.   Short-scale contrast equals low kilovoltage, high grid ratio, and high-speed screens. (Ref. 11, p. 145)

265. B.   An increase in kilovoltage produces a longer scale of contrast. The density would remain the same because 50 mAs at 65 kV is equal to 25 mAs at 75 kV. (Ref. 11, p. 122)

266. C.   Highest contrast or shortest scale equals low kilovoltage and highest ratio grid. (Ref. 11, p. 145)

267. B.   Short-scale contrast equals long OFD (air gap), high grid ratio, and low kilovoltage. (Ref. 11, p. 145)

268. B.   When using an FFD of 40 in, the structure to be examined would be placed at an OFD of 20 in, to result in a 2× magnification factor. (Ref. 11, p. 51)

269. A.   Total size distortion results from the combined effects of both OFD and FFD. (Ref. 11, p. 50)

270. B.   Since FFD also affects size distortion of the image, an increase in FFD can offset the size distortion occurring from the air gap. (Ref. 11, p. 50)

271. D.   Penumbra or unsharpness occurring from edge gradient is compared to a light beam casting a shadow on a wall as it relates to the x-ray beam recording the image on a film. (Ref. 6, p. 279)

272. A.   Distortion of the image occurs as the FFD is decreased. (Ref. 11, p. 50)

273. A. Geometric unsharpness is influenced by size of focus times OFD over FOD. (Ref. 11, p. 28)

274. C. Whole-body immobilizers, selected-part immobilizers, and position achievers and maintainers are effective immobilization devices. Distribution of fat reduces the effect on the radiograph. (Ref. 11, p. 12)

275. D. kVp is a radiographic quality and is unrelated to penumbra. (Ref. 11, p. 31)

276. D. Grid ratio, kVp, and field size all have a direct relationship on radiographic contrast. (Ref. 11, p. 145)

277. D. The most effective device for removing the amount of unwanted radiation directed towards the film is the radiographic grid. (Ref. 11, p. 145)

278. B. Image sharpness or decreased penumbra occurs with a decrease in SID, FFD. (Ref. 11, p. 31)

279. C. A 40-in, instead of the 72-in, SID causes size distortion of the chest. (Ref. 11, p. 32)

280. D. Radiographic detail is decreased because of patient motion. To control involuntary motion, use the fastest possible exposure time with appropriate mAs levels. (Ref. 11, p. 11)

281. A. The problem of voluntary motion control becomes obvious when you are confronted with an injured patient who cannot hold still. (Ref. 11, p. 11)

282. D. Changes in FFD affect magnification recorded detail and without technique compensation density. (Ref. 11, p. 36)

283. A. Geometric sharpness or sharpness of detail is dependent on SID, OID, and FSS. Changes in these factors can increase or decrease sharpness. (Ref. 11, p. 36)

284. B. Thermionic emission relates to the radiation quantity (mAs), which is a radiographic factor. (Ref. 11, p. 73)

285. D. In the PA position, the frontal bone is in close contact with the film, and the reduced OFD will preserve recorded detail. (Ref. 11, p. 31)

286. D. Recorded detail is affected by OFD, FFD, and focal spot size under the geometry category. (Ref. 11, p. 36)

287. C. The best detail is obtained by the slowest-speed screen, smallest FSS, longest FFD (SID), and shortest OFD. (Ref. 11, p. 36)

288. B. mAs relates to photographic qualities. (Ref. 11, p. 96)

289. D. Impaired definition or increase image unsharpness can occur from motion, increased OFD, and decreased FFD. (Ref. 11, p. 31)

290. D. As the size of the focus decreases, the effect of "blooming" of the focus also decreases. (Ref. 11, p. 30)

291. B. The size and thickness of the crystal layer in intensifying screen have an effect on definition. (Ref. 11, p. 23)

292. C. Changes in OFD have a dramatic effect on definition. (Ref. 11, p. 31)

293. C. Detail is dependent upon FFD and OFD, control of motion, speed of the screens, size of the focus, and film screen contact. The amount of thermionic emission is unrelated to detail. (Ref. 11, p. 36)

294. A. Definition relates to the sharpness of the image structure. (Ref. 11, p. 4)

295. D. Motion unsharpness that is involuntary, such as physiologic motion, is controlled by selection of a fast exposure time. (Ref. 11, p. 11)

296. A. The best definition is slow-speed screens and the smallest focal spot size. (Ref. 11, p. 36)

297. C. The shortest OFD will exhibit the best definition. (Ref. 11, p. 36)

298. D. This change will usually lose the effect of the small focal spot and decrease the definition. (Ref. 11, p. 29)

299. C. The greatest definition is fast exposure time (motion eliminated), short OFD, long FFD, and slow-speed screens. (Ref. 11, p. 36)

300. A. Lack of penumbra limits geometric unsharpness and produces an image sharp in detail. Penumbra reduces resolution. (Ref. 6, p. 279)

301. D. The best recorded detail is fast exposure time, long SID, and short OFD. (Ref. 11, p. 36)

302. D. The greatest definition is longest SID and slowest-speed screens. (Ref. 11, p. 12)

303. B. The greatest recorded detail is fast exposure time, small focal spot size, long SID, and short OFD. (Ref. 11, p. 36)

304. A. The greatest density is high mAs, high kilovoltage, and low grid ratio. (Ref. 11, p. 96)

305. D. 450 mA at 0.66; 1,200 mA at 0.25 sec; and 600 mA at 0.50 sec are all combinations of 300 mAs. (Ref. 11, p. 96)

306. B. When the 15% rule, screen intensification factors, and the mAs/distance relationship are used, all three techniques are equal. (Ref. 11, p. 96)

307. D. An mAs change of at least 30% is required to produce a noticeable change in density. 40 to 60 mAs = 50%. (Ref. 11, p. 78)

308. D. mAs = mA × time; 200 × 1/4 = 50 mAs and 500 × 1/10 = 50 mAs. (Ref. 11, p. 96)

309. B.
$$\frac{300}{x} = \frac{6 \ (16{:}1)}{4 \ (8{:}1)}$$
$$6x = 1,200$$
$$x = 200$$
1/40 sec high-speed screens = 1/20 sec par-speed. (Ref. 11, p. 144)

310. B. The greatest density is high mAs, short SID, and low grid ratio. (Ref. 11, p. 96)

311. B. From 100 to 300 mA more electrons will be boiled off the filament, with more photons produced. (Ref. 11, p. 73)

312. B. $300 \times 10 = 30$ mAs. The 15% rule states that you increase your kVp by 15% and you compensate for this by a reduction of mAs by one-half.

$$\frac{1}{2} \times 2 = \frac{1}{4} \qquad \frac{30}{1} \times \frac{1}{4} = 7.5 \text{ mAs}$$

(Ref. 11, p. 82)

313. D. 100 mAs at 70 kV equals 1200 mA times 1/6 sec, or 200 mAs at 60 kV. (Ref. 11, p. 96)

314. D. The fastest exposure time would be needed to control motion. (Ref. 11, p. 15)

315. D. Highest mAs (mA × time) equals greatest number of photons. (Ref. 11, p. 96)

316. C. $300 \times 1/12 = 25$ and

$$\frac{400}{25} = 1/16 \qquad \text{(Ref. 11, p. 74)}$$

317. B. High-speed screens are approximately twice as fast as par-speed screens. 20 mAs par equals 10 mAs high. 200 mA at 1/20 sec equals 10 mAs. (Ref. 11, p. 86)

318. D. $\dfrac{60 \text{ mAs}}{x} = \dfrac{40^2}{30^2} = 33.75$ mAs, or 34 mAs

(Ref. 11, p. 79)

319. B. 1/30 sec (TT) × 5 (12:1) = 5/30, or 1/6 sec. (Ref. 11, p. 144)

320. D. The highest density is high mAs, high kilovoltage, and low grid ratio. (Ref. 11, p. 96)

321. C. A 5-cm increase in size can be adjusted by 2 × mA or exposure time, or a 15% increase in kilovoltage. (Ref. 11, p. 144)

322. A. kVp/mAs relationship: 100 to 200 mAs can be compensated for by a reduction of 15% kVp. 80 − 12 (15% of 80) = 68 kVp. (Ref. 11, p. 82)

323. D. Higher kVp results in greater scatter radiation, for it alters beam quality and the penetrating ability of the beam. (Ref. 11, p. 117)

324. B. $\dfrac{80 \text{ mAs}}{1,000 \text{ mA}} = 0.08$ sec
(Ref. 11, p. 75)

325. B. 50 msec, or one twentieth of a second, can be 0.05 sec decimal or 1/20 sec fraction values. (Ref. 11, p. 76)

326. B. 50 mAs at 80 kV is equal to 100 mAs at 70 kV. (Ref. 11, p. 81)

327. B. 100 mA at 1/2 sec, and 200 mA at 1/4, both yield 50 mAs. (Ref. 11, p. 75)

328. B. 100 mA, 1/20 sec = 5 mAs. From TT to 10:1 grid = 5 × original mAs. 200 × 1/8 = 25 mAs. (Ref. 11, p. 144)

329. C. A film with the most density has high mAs, kilovoltage, and screens. (Ref. 11, p. 96)

330. C. mA × time = mAs. Most mAs equals most density. (Ref. 11, p. 75)

331. B. 200 mA × 1/2 sec = 100 mAs. 500 mA × 0.2 sec = 100 mAs. (Ref. 11, p. 75)

332. B. 100 mA × 1 sec × 80 kV = 8,000 HU adjusted to 100 mA × 1/2 sec × 80 kV = 4,500 HU. 8,000 − 4,500 = 3,500 HU less with the adjusted technique. (Ref. 29, p. 230)

333. D. A film with the least density has low mAs, kilovoltage, and long SID. (Ref. 11, p. 96)

334. B. The greatest density is the highest mAs related to kilovoltage, screen speed, and FFD. (Ref. 11, p. 96)

335. C. A change of 60 to 70 kV, par- to high-speed screens, and 200 to 400 mAs all will double the radiographic density. A change in focal spot size can only affect density if the mA also changes. (Ref. 11, p. 96)

336. D. 300 mA multiplied by 100 msec, 1/10 sec, or 0.1 sec all equal 30 mAs. (Ref. 11, p. 74)

337. B. 300 × x = 15.   x = 0.05 sec. (Ref. 11, p. 75)

338. A. Collimation minimizes secondary radiation, thus decreasing the density and increasing the contrast. (Ref. 11, p. 145)

339. A. A change in overall technique of 35% to 50% is required to see any visible change in density. A 30% change in mAs is considered minimal. (Ref. 11, p. 78)

340. D. Focal spot size is strictly geometrical, and has nothing to do with x-ray output. Choices A, B, and C would roughly double image density. (Ref. 11)

341. B. 200 mA × 0.10 sec = 400 mA at 0.05 sec. (Ref. 11, p. 96)

342. A. A change of at least 30% in mAs is required. 200 mA × 4/5 sec = 160 mAs and 3 kV more. (Ref. 11, p. 78)

343. C. From 20 to 10 mAs is equal to 64 kVp, up 15% to 73 kVp. (Ref. 11, p. 75)

344. A. A reduction in exposure time is the most important method in the control of physiologic motion. (Ref. 11, p. 15)

345. D. The fastest exposure time will decrease the chance of motion unsharpness. (Ref. 11, p. 11)

346. C. A faster exposure time will decrease the motion factor and help maintain sharp definition. (Ref. 11, p. 11)

347. B. 1,000 mA × 0.07 sec = 70 mAs. (Ref. 11, p. 75)

348. B. 15% of 46 kV = 7 kV. (Ref. 11, p. 81)

349. C.   1. $\dfrac{60}{x} = \dfrac{80 \text{ in}}{40 \text{ in}} = \dfrac{2^2}{1^2} = \dfrac{4}{1}$

2. $15 \text{ mAs} = \dfrac{1 \text{ (nongrid)}}{3 \text{ (6:1 grid)}}$

3. $45 \text{ mAs} \div 2 = 22.5 \text{ mAs}$. $70 \text{ kV} + 10 \, (15\%) = 80 \text{ kV}$. (Ref. 11, p. 96)

350. A. In long scale or high contrast, the recorded densities are quite different from one another. (Ref. 11, p. 121)

351. C. Shorter wavelength radiation is generated by higher kilovoltage, and produces greater penetrating ability. (Ref. 11, p. 87)

352. B. Fog is reduced when the object is moved farther from the film and, therefore, contrast is increased with a fog reduction. (Ref. 11, p. 126)

353. C. The nongrid technique would have the greatest effect on density and contrast. (Ref. 11, p. 144)

354. B. Milliamperage is unrelated to subject contrast that results from different absorption characteristics of the structure making up the part. (Ref. 11, p. 112)

355. B. The quantity of radiation needed with thick body parts to produce the desired density adds to the problems of scattered radiation that can be corrected by employment of a high-ratio grid. (Ref. 11, p. 143)

356. C. 100 kV + 15% (15% rule) = 115 kV. (Ref. 11, p. 81)

357. A. Resolution is usually identified as the number of line pairs per millimeter the system is capable of recording. (Ref. 11, p. 18)

358. C. Kilovoltage influences the radiographic density of the image. The influence is indirect because kilovoltage is a variable. A change of 15% of the kilovoltage will approximately double or cut in half the original density. (Ref. 11, p. 81)

359. D. By going up 20 kV, you would alter film latitude, patient absorption, and wavelengths. (Ref. 11, p. 87)

360. D. The impact of subject contrast on radiographic contrast becomes evident when you consider the multiplicity of different tissues, together with their different thicknesses and opacities, within every body part. (Ref. 11, p. 113)

361. C. Intensifying screens inherently produce an image with a higher scale of contrast compared to a similar procedure performed without screens. Contrast increases as screen speed increases. (Ref. 11, p. 145)

362. D. A change from 86 kV to 80 kV is equal to an exposure time change of 1/2 sec to 3/4 sec. (Ref. 11, p. 96)

363. D. OFD is the factor that is most critical in consideration of geometric unsharpness. (Ref. 11, p. 33)

364. B. 85 kVp is too much to penetrate a normal child's lateral skull. (Ref. 11, p. 123)

365. D. Both OFD and FFD (SID) affect size distortion. Poor alignment of the object to the focus and film will cause shape distortion. (Ref. 11, p. 54)

366. B.
$$\frac{20}{x} = \frac{72}{56} \qquad \frac{9^2}{7^2} = \frac{81}{49}$$
$$81x = 980$$
$$x = 12.10 \ (12) \ \text{mAs}$$
(Ref. 11, p. 79)

367. C. A change from 24 in to 48 in equals a fourfold change from the original mAs. A change in screen speed is equivalent to doubling the mAs. The kilovoltage would have to change twice with the 15% rule. (Ref. 11, p. 96)

368. B. Geometric unsharpness or penumbra reduces resolution and is undesirable. (Ref. 6, p. 279)

369. C. 300 mA at 1/5 sec = 60 mAs (80 mR). 400 mA at 1/3 sec = 120 mAs (160 mR). (Ref. 29, p. 63)

370. D. A change from 40 to 20 in results in a fourfold change in the mAs delivered to the film, which is compensated for by using an 8:1 grid. (Ref. 11, p. 144)

371. A. A change in distance from 200 cm to 100 cm requires a change to one-fourth of the original exposure time, from 0.1 sec to 0.025 sec. (Ref. 11, p. 79)

372. B. 2/10 at 80 in = 1/20 at 40 in. (Ref. 11, p. 79)

373. A. $\dfrac{100}{x} = \dfrac{40}{30} = \dfrac{4^2}{3^2} = \dfrac{16}{9}$
$16x = 900$
$x = 56.25$ mAs. (Ref. 11, p. 79)

374. B. This change would produce approximately five times less in mAs required, since no adjustment was made for TT to 10:1 grid. (Ref. 11, p. 144)

375. C. $\dfrac{75}{x} = \dfrac{2\ (5{:}1\ \text{grid})}{4\ (8{:}1\ \text{grid})} = 150$ mAs
(Ref. 11, p. 144)

376. D. TT to 12:1 grid = 5 × 1/5 sec = 1 sec. (Ref. 11, p. 144)

377. B. $\dfrac{120}{x} = \dfrac{5\ (10{:}1\ \text{grid})}{3\ (6{:}1\ \text{grid})} = 360 \div 5 = 72$ mAs
(Ref. 11, p. 144)

378. C. $\dfrac{100}{x} = \dfrac{4\ (8{:}1\ \text{grid})}{2\ (5{:}1\ \text{grid})} = 200$ mAs
$4x = 200$ mAs.
$x = 50$ mAs. 90 kVp to 80 kVp = 50 mAs to 100 mAs. (Ref. 11, p. 144)

379. D. $\dfrac{100}{x} = \dfrac{5\ (12{:}1\ \text{grid})}{3\ (6{:}1\ \text{grid})}$

$5x = 300$

$x = 60$

If 90 kVp goes to 76, then 60 mAs goes to 120 mAs. (Ref. 11, p. 144)

380. B. 75 kVp to 86 kVp = 80 mAs to 40 mAs.

$\dfrac{40}{x} = \dfrac{1\ (\text{nongrid})}{3\ (6{:}1\ \text{grid})}$

$x = 120$ mAs

(Ref. 11, p. 144)

381. B. 200 mA, 0.03 sec with par-speed screens is equal to 200 mA, 0.015 high-speed screens. (Ref. 11, p. 96)

382. A. Quantum mottle is a phenomenon occurring from rapid imaging systems and reduced radiation. (Ref. 11, p. 24)

383. B. Poor film screen contact will result in an increased level of image unsharpness in those areas experiencing poor contact. (Ref. 11, p. 25)

384. C. To compensate from par- to high-speed screens, use 50% less exposure time from 0.03 to 0.015 sec. (Ref. 11, p. 96)

385. D. The latent image is that visible image produced in the film emulsion by light or x-rays, which is changed to a visible or manifest image during development. (Ref. 29, p. 318)

386. B. In practice, an acceptable base-plus-fog density for fresh film is approximately 0.18, which means that the inherent chemical fog is about 0.04. (Ref. 35, p. 41)

387. B. A 20-in (50-cm) air gap provides cleanup of scattered radiation as well as a 15 ratio grid. Therefore, a high kilovoltage can be used without excessive fog on the radiograph. (Ref. 29, p. 377)

388. D. Secondary radiation refers to those x-ray photons that have undergone a change in direction after interacting with atoms. Body thickness, tissue density, and kilovoltage will all affect the level of secondary radiation. (Ref. 29, p. 184)

389. A.   The latent image is the visible image produced in the film emulsion by light or x-rays, which is changed to a manifest image during development. (Ref. 29, p. 318)

390. B.   Two types of devices are available to reduce the amount of scattered radiation. They are beam restrictors and grid; filters do not affect scatter. (Ref. 6, p. 187)

391. D.   The number of grid strips or grid lines per inch is called the grid frequency. (Ref. 6, p. 198)

392. D.   A grid is required for anatomical parts greater than 12-cm thick and kilovoltage values above 65. (Ref. 11, p. 142)

393. D.   Beam limitation is the primary technique to employ in your attempt to reduce radiographic fog. (Ref. 11, p. 131)

394. C.   The grid significantly improves the visibility of the image. It does not reduce patient exposure. (Ref. 11, p. 142)

395. B.   Generally, as the grid ratio increases, the efficiency of the grid also increases. (Ref. 11, p. 140)

396. D.   Grid ratio is one of the physical attributes of a grid and is a major influence on grid efficiency. (Ref. 11, p. 140)

397. C.   Collimation restricts the size of the primary beam and is the best technique to employ in reducing radiographic fog. (Ref. 11, p. 131)

398. D. $4.0 \div 0.25 = 16$. (Ref. 11, p. 140)

399. B.   Most grids are linear in design. The lead strips are designed to extend in the same direction and are recorded as a linear pattern on the film. (Ref. 11, p. 134)

400. B.   Grid ratio deals with three important dimensions on a grid: the thickness of the grid material, the thickness of the interspace material, and the height of the grid. The grid ratio is the height divided by the interspace thickness. (Ref. 6, p. 198)

401. B. The grid is designed to transmit only those x-rays whose direction is on a line from the source to the image receptor. (Ref. 6, p. 197)

402. D. Barium spills will cause artifacts of low density on the radiograph. (Ref. 33, p. 328)

403. D. The changes in tissue thickness in the femur require proper utilization of the anode heel effect to ensure an even distribution of film density. (Ref. 11, p. 97)

404. D. The anode heel effect will change as the focal spot of the x-ray tube changes, along with the FFD employed and field size. (Ref. 6, p. 118)

405. A. Filtration alters beam quality and exposure rate. It does not affect radiographic definition. (Ref. 29, p. 172)

406. D. Geometric unsharpness factors include focal spot size, OFD, FFD (SID). Body part size does not influence geometric unsharpness. (Ref. 11, p. 29)

407. C. Greater penetration occurs when the kVp is increased. (Ref. 6, p. 177)

408. D. Changes in kilovoltage or the quality factor of the beam will alter latitude, patient absorption, and wavelengths. (Ref. 11, p. 81)

409. B. Heavy film cartons should be stored and transported on edge to prevent pressure marks. (Ref. 33, p. 50)

410. C. When silver bromide halides are struck by light or x-rays, the crystals undergo an electrochemical change in the formation of the latent image. (Ref. 29, p. 318)

411. C. By absorbing light, the dye or "tinting" reduces screen unsharpness, while simultaneously reducing film density. (Ref. 35, p. 67)

412. D. The most predominant interaction of x-rays in the energy range of diagnostic radiology is by way of photoelectric effect. Bone with an effective Z = 20 experiences more photoelectric interaction than soft tissue with an effective Z = 12. Hence, contrast is achieved. (Ref. 6, p. 163)

413. B. Compared with untinted film, this coloring results in less eyestrain and fatigue for the radiologist and, therefore, is conducive to more efficient and accurate diagnosis. (Ref. 6, p. 213)

414. C. The visible image (manifest) is obtained by development of the film and its conversion to black metallic silver. (Ref. 6, p. 215)

415. B. Phototimer cassettes have a radiolucent back to permit the radiation reaching the film to continue on the automatic exposure control. (Ref. 35, p. 62)

416. B. The protective coating closest to the film is 15- to 25-μm thick and is applied to the face of the screen to make it resistant to abrasion and damage caused by handling. (Ref. 6, p. 241)

417. C. Some newer and rare-earth phosphors are barium strontium sulfate, barium fluorochloride, gadolinium, lanthanum, and lanthanum oxybromide. (Ref. 29, p. 300)

418. D. The three factors influencing material unsharpness are the type of radiographic film, the use of intensifying screens, and the film screen contact. (Ref. 11, p. 16)

419. B. Poor screen contact causes a blurred image or loss of definition. (Ref. 29, p. 303)

420. B. The 1-mm base can be made of high-grade cardboard, polyester, or metal. Polyester meets the requirements for base material. (Ref. 6, p. 243)

421. A. The speed or intensification factor is the ratio of the exposure required without screens to the exposure required with screens to get the same degree of film blackening. (Ref. 29, p. 298)

Explanatory Answers / 133

422. B. Two types of luminescence occur with certian crystals: emission of light by fluorescence and delayed emission of light by phosphorescence. (Ref. 29, p. 296)

423. C. The emulsion consists of a homogeneous mixture of gelatin and silver halide crystals. (Ref. 6, p. 214)

424. B. Osteolysis would be considered an atrophic condition requiring a reduction in normal exposure factors. (Ref. 11, p. 71)

425. C. Carbon dioxide and air are gases that are the least dense body substances. (Ref. 11, p. 115)

426. A. Bone is the most dense naturally occurring tissue within the body and absorbs a greater percentage of radiation than any other body tissue. (Ref. 11, p. 116)

427. B. Double the mAs for increased part thickness and increase the kVp by 10% for increased part opacity. (Ref. 11, p. 97)

428. D. When patients with involuntary motion causing conditions are radiographed, you should reduce exposure time as much as possible. (Ref. 11, p. 11)

429. C. Density of cast = 2 × mAs + 10% kVp. (Ref. 11, p. 92)

430. D. Changes in the thickness of the body part (atrophy) may require the technologist to change the quantity or quality of radiation, or both. (Ref. 11, p. 71)

431. A. Osteomalacia is a destructive (easy to penetrate) pathology. (Ref. 35, p. 240)

432. B. The application of compression bands may cause a considerable change in the thickness of the part to be radiographed. (Ref. 35, p. 238)

433. D. Emphysema is a destructive pathological condition requiring a reduction in normal exposure factors. (Ref. 35, p. 240)

434. B. The presence of significant fluid or ascites means more scattered/secondary radiation fog. (Ref. 35, p. 247)

435. B. Voluntary motion can be controlled by careful explanation of the procedure, immobilization devices, and fast exposure times. (Ref. 11, p. 10)

436. B. Multiple myeloma is a destructive pathological condition requiring a reduction in exposure factors. (Ref. 35, p. 241)

437. D. Empyema is an additive hard-to-penetrate respiratory pathology requiring increased exposure factors. (Ref. 35, p. 241)

438. B. Active tuberculosis is a destructive (easy to penetrate) condition. (Ref. 35, p. 241)

439. A. With osteoporosis, there is a loss of calcium from the bone, leaving it less dense. Emphysema is a destructive lung disease that is also easily penetrated. (Ref. 35, p. 241)

440. B. The combination of hydroquinone and metol assure optimum development of the radiographic image. (Ref. 29, p. 323)

441. D. Potassium bromide is an antifog agent that keeps the unexposed crystals from being chemically attacked. (Ref. 6, p. 227)

442. B. The developer consists of solvents: developing agents, accelerators, preservatives, restrainers, and hardeners. (Ref. 29, p. 323)

443. D. Potassium bromide and potassium iodide are used as restrainers or antifoggants. Bromide ions protect unexposed grains from the action of the developer to minimize fog growth. (Ref. 29, p. 323)

444. D. The primary function of the transport system is to move the film through the processor at a precisely controlled speed. The rollers produce solution agitation and the last few rollers act as a squeegee. (Ref. 26, p. 98)

445. C. The function of the developer and fixer is to convert the latent image to a visible image by means of various solutions. (Ref. 29, p. 323)

446. C. The hardener made of chrome alum or potassium alum "tans" or hardens the gelatin in the emulsion, thereby protecting it against scratches. (Ref. 29, p. 327)

447. D. The crossover rack is a small rack located between the developer and fixer and is composed of rollers and guide shoes. (Ref. 6, p. 233)

448. D. In order to shorten processing times within the various sections, hydroquinone and phenidone are the developing agents, along with cycon, which retards oxidation. (Ref. 29, p. 333)

449. B. With optimum time and temperature being 68° at 5 min, and applying the formula of 2° equals plus or minus 1/2 min, at 72° or +4° equals −1 min. (Ref. 16, p. 102)

450. B. The fixer solution consists of solvent, clearing agent, preservative, hardener, acidifier, and buffer. (Ref. 16, p. 95)

4 Radiographic Procedures

The major subject areas covered in radiographic procedures include the following.

1. Anatomical nomenclature, body cavities, division of the body, positioning terminology, and topographical anatomy, including surface markings and prominences.
2. Positioning aids; immobilization devices; breathing instructions; patient preparation; handling of the seriously ill, pediatric, geriatric, and difficult patients; and various radiographic pathologies.
3. The various projections, anatomical structures, diseases, and conditions of the skeletal system that relate to the
   a. shoulder girdle and upper extremity
   b. pelvis, hip joint, and lower extremity
   c. vertebral column
   d. thorax
   e. skull, facial bones, sinuses, and mastoids
   f. joints and articulations
4. The anatomical structures, diseases, and conditions that affect the various body systems with emphasis on the
   a. circulatory system
   b. respiratory system
   c. digestive system
   d. urinary system
   e. reproductive system
   f. nervous system
5. Common contrast media studies of the
   a. gastrointestinal tract

    b. biliary tract
    c. genitourinary tract
    d. related body systems
6. Special radiographic procedures of
    a. angiography
    b. arthrography
    c. myelography
    d. pacemaker
    e. mammography
    f. tomography
    g. cardiovascular

DIRECTIONS (Questions 451–700): Each of the questions or incomplete statements below is followed by four suggested answers or completions. Select the **one** that is best in each case.

451. Which of the following baselines is important when doing a PA skull radiograph?
    A. Orbitomeatal
    B. Supraorbitomeatal
    C. Mentomeatal
    D. Glabellomeatal

452. Which of the following are vertical planes that pass through the body from front to back, dividing it into right and left portions?
    1. Parasagittal
    2. Coronal plane
    3. Sagittal
    A. 1 and 2 only
    B. 1 and 3 only
    C. 2 and 3 only
    D. 1, 2, and 3

453. The superior medial portion of the abdomen is known as the
    A. epigastrium
    B. hypogastrium
    C. paragastrium
    D. hypergastrium

454. An x-ray taken of the extremities in abduction means that it is
    A. fixed in its natural position
    B. moved toward the midline of the body
    C. rotated internally
    D. drawn away from the midline of the body

455. When a part of the body is examined in eversion, this means that the part is
  A. rotated outward
  B. in natural position
  C. rotated inward
  D. abducted from the body

456. The angle between the eyelids is called the
  A. acanthion
  B. glabella
  C. nasion
  D. canthus

457. The smooth, round prominence above the root of the nose is called the
  A. nasion
  B. canthus
  C. glabella
  D. inion

458. Which of the following is considered part of the ventral body cavity?
    1. Thoracic cavity
    2. Abdominopelvic cavity
    3. Cranial cavity
  A. 1 and 2 only
  B. 1 and 3 only
  C. 2 and 3 only
  D. 1, 2, and 3

459. The stomach is located primarily within the
  A. right lower quadrant (RLQ)
  B. right upper quadrant (RUQ)
  C. left upper quadrant (LUQ)
  D. left lower quadrant (LLQ)

460. Which of the following is located within the RUQ of the body?
  A. Duodenal cap
  B. Descending colon
  C. Appendix
  D. Splenic flexure

461. Which of the following organs is located in the hypogastric region?
  A. Spleen
  B. Gallbladder
  C. Urinary bladder
  D. Vermiform appendix

462. Which of the following organs is located in the right hypochondriac region?
  A. Spleen
  B. Gallbladder
  C. Urinary bladder
  D. Appendix

463. Which of the following structures is **MOST** anterior?
  A. Gallbladder
  B. Hepatic ducts (right and left)
  C. Common bile duct
  D. Common hepatic duct

464. The xiphisternal junction is at the level of
  A. D-6
  B. D-9
  C. D-12
  D. L-2

465. If a patient measures 22 cm in the PA position for a chest, and 34 cm in the lateral position, what would he/she measure in a true oblique?
  A. 18 cm
  B. 25 cm
  C. 28 cm
  D. 31 cm

466. Between which vertebrae are the kidneys normally found?
A. D-6 and D-8
B. D-9 and D-11
C. D-12 and L-3
D. L-4 and L-5

467. The hypersthenic habitus is a build that is
A. extremely slender
B. massive
C. slender
D. normal

468. There are four distinct body types. Which of the following is the **MOST** common?
A. Hyposthenic
B. Sthenic
C. Hypersthenic
D. Asthenic

469. Legg-Calvé-Perthes disease would be demonstrated on a radiography of the
A. knee
B. pelvis
C. tibial tuberosity
D. ankle

470. In which of the following body types is the gallbladder **MOST** superior?
A. Hyposthenic
B. Hypersthenic
C. Sthenic
D. Ectomorphic

471. Dysplasia refers to
A. impairment of speech
B. abnormal development of tissue
C. malposition
D. difficult breathing

472. Which of the following conditions occurs primarily as a childhood ailment?
    A. Ewing's sarcoma
    B. Paget's disease
    C. Osteoporosis
    D. Osteoarthritis

473. What term is applied to an organ that **NEVER** develops?
    A. Hypoplasia
    B. Agenesis
    C. Hypertrophy
    D. Dysplasia

474. The spread of malignant tumor cells from the primary tumor to another tissue(s) in the body is
    A. neoplasm
    B. hyperplasia
    C. metastasis
    D. invasion

475. Which statement is **INCORRECT**?
    A. Rickets is a metabolic bone disease
    B. Osteopetrosis is a marble bone disease
    C. Impaction relates to a bone that is splintered
    D. Dextrocardia relates to the heart on the right side of the thorax

476. Which statement relating to disease is **INCORRECT**?
    A. Ewing's sarcoma is a malignant neoblastic disease
    B. Hodgkin's disease is a benign condition
    C. Paget's disease is also known as osteitis deformans
    D. Wilms' tumor originates in the kidney

477. An abnormal **DECREASE** in bone density due to failure of the osteoblasts to produce bone that is quite common in postmenopausal women is called
    A. osteoporosis
    B. osteomyelitis
    C. osteoitis
    D. osteosarcoma

144 / Radiography

478. Which of the following statements relating to fractures is **INCOR-RECT?**

   A. Comminuted fractures occur when the bone is broken into several pieces

   B. Colle's fractures involve the distal end of the ulna

   C. Pott's fractures involve the distal end of the fibula

   D. Greenstick fractures occur in children

479. Which statement is **INCORRECT?**

   A. Large relates to macro

   B. Tumor relates to oma

   C. Para relates to around

   D. Ectomy relates to cut out

480. A sudden loss of consciousness followed by paralysis is called

   A. apolepsis

   B. apoplexy

   C. apoptosis

   D. aposia

481. A fracture that involves the pulling loose of bone by aligament or tendon is called

   A. an oblique fracture

   B. a fatigue facture

   C. a Colle's fracture

   D. an avulsion fracture

482. Inflammation of bone, especially the marrow, is called

   A. osteogenesis

   B. osteomyelitis

   C. osteoneuralgia

   D. osteochondritis

483. Which of the following conditions occurs from a calcium and vitamin D deficiency?

   A. Infantile osteomalacia

   B. Scurvy

   C. Multiple myeloma

   D. Gargoylism

484. Which of the following fracture types is unrelated to the others?
A. Stress
B. March
C. Tripod
D. Insufficiency

485. A tumor composed of both cartilaginous and bony substance is an
A. osteosarcoma
B. osteoblastoma
C. osteocystoma
D. osteochondroma

486. The degenerative disease where the walls of the arteries lose elasticity from hardening is known as
A. atherosclerosis
B. arterionecrosis
C. athetosis
D. artheriostenosis

487. A disease of unknown or obscure cause is said to be
A. systemic
B. pseudopathic
C. epidemic
D. idiopathic

488. A spontaneous fracture would be associated with
A. pathology
B. crepitus
C. trauma
D. metabolism

489. Which of the following contrast materials is routinely used for arthrography?
1. Air
2. Oily iodine compounds (such as Pantopaque)
3. Aqueous iodine compounds (such as Renografin)
A. 1 and 2 only
B. 1 and 3 only
C. 2 and 3 only
D. 1, 2, and 3

490. Which of the following is an aqueous contrast material that is used for myelography?
A. Pantopaque
B. Ethiodol
C. Hypaque
D. Amipaque

491. $BaSO_4$ is considered a
A. cholecystogogue
B. suspension contrast media
C. biliary stimulant
D. cholecystokinin

492. A contrast media commonly used in lymphography is
A. Renografin
B. Cholografin
C. Ethiodol
D. Amipaque

493. Which of the following is a normal occurrence during the injection of iodine contrast medias for intravenous urography?
1. A hot flush feeling in the face
2. Excessive urticaria
3. A metallic taste in the mouth
A. 1 and 2 only
B. 1 and 3 only
C. 2 and 3 only
D. 1, 2, and 3

494. During retrograde urography, the amount of contrast media usually injected into the renal pelvis is
A. 1 to 2 cc
B. 3 to 5 cc
C. 7 to 10 cc
D. 15 to 20 cc

495. The amount of contrast media used to fill the uterine cavity during hysterosalpingography is approximately
A. 4 mL
B. 6 to 8 mL
C. 10 mL
D. 15 to 20 mL

496. The contrast material used in pneumoarthrography is a(an)
A. aqueous opaque medium
B. gaseous medium
C. air and aqueous opaque medium
D. oily opaque medium

497. The contrast media **MOST** commonly used in IV cholangiography is
A. Telepaque
B. Diodrast
C. Lipiodol
D. Cholografin

498. Which of the following is **NOT** considered a contrast media for oral cholecystography?
A. Oragrafin
B. Meglumine
C. Cholografin
D. Bilopaque

499. Which of the following contrast media matched to anatomical parts is **INCORRECT**?
A. Sodium ditrizoid for kidneys
B. Hypaque 50% for lymphangiography
C. Conray 60% for cerebral angiography
D. Renografin 60% for renal angiography

500. In hip-nailing radiography, the position of the patient resembles the
A. Holmblad position
B. Danielus-Miller method
C. Ottonello method
D. Pearson projection

501. In order to minimize the hazard of blood clots when performing cardiovascular investigations, which of the following is usually coated around the guide wire and catheter?
A. Phentolamine
B. Heparin
C. Procaine
D. Adrenalin

502. Which of the following carpal bones articulates with the first digit?
A. Pisiform
B. Hamate
C. Trapezoid
D. Trapezium

503. When a bilateral examination of the hands is requested, rotation distortion can be avoided if the hands are
A. separately positioned
B. positioned at the radiographer's discretion
C. simultaneously positioned
D. supinated

504. Which bones are **BEST** visualized in the carpal canal position?
1. Pisiform
2. Lunate
3. Hamate
A. 1 and 2 only
B. 1 and 3 only
C. 2 and 3 only
D. 1, 2, and 3

505. Which of the following carpals is **NOT** involved with the wrist joint?
   A. Capitate
   B. Scaphoid
   C. Triangular
   D. Lunate

506. The first carpometacarpal joint is the articulation of the first metacarpal bone and the
   A. lunate
   B. greater multangular
   C. pisiform
   D. triangular

507. When radiographing the elbow joint in the lateral position, it is necessary to flex the elbow
   A. 20°
   B. 35°
   C. 60°
   D. 90°

508. Which of the following positions will **BEST** demonstrate the coronoid process of the elbow?
   A. Medial oblique
   B. Flexion with a 10° cephalic tube angle
   C. Lateral
   D. Oblique external rotation

509. Which position of the elbow will clearly demonstrate the "fat pad" sign?
   A. Lateral oblique
   B. Lateral
   C. Anterioposterior
   D. Medial oblique

510. The anatomical neck of the numerus lies
  A. inferior to the surgical neck
  B. superior to the tuberosities
  C. superior to the head of the humerus
  D. inferior to the diaphysis

511. Which of the following is the **MOST** superior?
  A. Trochlea
  B. Olecranon process
  C. Radial notch
  D. Capitulum

512. Which portion of the humerus does the semilunar notch articulate with?
  A. Coronoid process
  B. Capitellum
  C. Trochlea
  D. Lateral condyle

513. A bony prominence found in the region of the shoulder would be the process of the
  A. acromion
  B. coronoid
  C. styloid
  D. olecranon

514. The bicipital groove is located on the
  A. scapula
  B. clavicle
  C. radius
  D. humerus

515. The humerus articulates with the ulna on the medial side at the
  A. coronoid fossa
  B. capitellum
  C. glenoid fossa
  D. trochlea

516. Which position of the shoulder will clearly demonstrate the greater tuberosity?
  A. Internal rotation
  B. Transaxillary
  C. Neutral position
  D. External rotation

517. The central ray for an AP shoulder, nontrauma, should be directed to the
  A. coracoid process
  B. glenoid fossa
  C. acromion
  D. acromioclavicular joint

518. Which of the following positions should **NEVER** be used when a fracture or dislocation of the shoulder is suspected?
  A. Anteroposterior (neutral position)
  B. Transaxillary
  C. Transthoracic lateral
  D. Anteroposterior erect

519. Which of the following statements is **INCORRECT?**
  A. The trochlea is located on the humerus
  B. The manubrium is part of the sternum
  C. The acromion is the most prominent point of the shoulder
  D. The glenoid fossa is part of the humerus

520. The transthoracic lateral position (Lawrence method) is used for demonstration of the
  A. scapula
  B. clavicle
  C. elbow
  D. proximal humerus

521. Which of the following does **NOT** apply to the transthoracic projection of the shoulder?
    A. It demonstrates proximal humerus superimposed by lung field
    B. It can be used to demonstrate joint pathology such as arthritis
    C. A long exposure time is utilized
    D. The affected side is closest to the film

522. The process of the scapula which is **MOST** anterior is the
    A. coracoid
    B. acromion
    C. coronoid
    D. glenoid

523. A patient has tenderness and swelling at the base of the fifth metatarsal. Which of the following positions will **BEST** help rule out a fracture in that area?
    A. AP with a straight central ray
    B. AP with a 15° cephalic tilt of the central ray
    C. Medial oblique
    D. External oblique

524. The dorsoplantar projection of the foot will clearly demonstrate the joint spaces between the metatarsals and midfoot if the tube is angled
    A. 5° anterior
    B. 10° posterior
    C. 15° anterior
    D. 20° posterior

525. The tarsal that lies just anterior to the talus is the
    A. navicular
    B. calcaneous
    C. cuboid
    D. first cuniform

526. The axial plantodorsal projection of the calcaneus requires a tube angulation of
    A. 10°
    B. 25°
    C. 40°
    D. 54°

527. Which position of the foot will show the **MOST** anatomy free of superimposition?
    A. AP
    B. Lateral
    C. Plantodorsal
    D. Oblique

528. In the oblique projection, the foot is rotated
    A. 15° internally
    B. 60° externally
    C. 90° from AP
    D. 45° internally

529. The AP projection of the ankle does **NOT** demonstrate the
    A. upper portion of the astragalus
    B. inferior tibiofibular articulation
    C. distal tibia and fibula
    D. ankle joint

530. In order to demonstrate the upper portion of the astragalus properly, which of the following projections is used?
    A. Dorsoplantar foot
    B. Medial oblique foot
    C. Oblique lateral ankle
    D. AP ankle

531. The 45° medial oblique projection of the ankle will clearly demonstrate the
    A. talocalcaneal articulation
    B. lateral malleolus
    C. metatarso-phalangeal joints
    D. trochlear process

532. To insure a true lateral position of the lower leg you would check the
1. malleoli of the tibia and fibula
2. epicondyles of the femur
3. rotation of the affected leg
   A. 1 and 2 only
   B. 1 and 3 only
   C. 2 and 3 only
   D. 1, 2, and 3

533. Which of the following projections of the knee **BEST** demonstrates the head of the fibula?
   A. Anterolateral oblique
   B. Anteromedial oblique
   C. Camp-coventry
   D. Anteroposterior

534. In relationship to the anatomical position, which statement is **CORRECT**?
   A. The radius is medial to the ulna
   B. The third metacarpal is lateral to the second metacarpal
   C. The fibula is medial to the tibia
   D. The third metatarsal is lateral to the second metatarsal

535. When radiographing the knee in the lateral projection, the patellar surface can be clearly demonstrated by
   A. axial flexion of 45°
   B. slightly flexing the knee
   C. angling the tube 35° to 40°
   D. flexion of approximately 30°

536. The knee joint is topographically located as a point which is
   A. inferior to the patellar apex
   B. inferior to the patellar base
   C. superior to the patellar apex
   D. superior to the patellar base

537. The tunnel (Holmblad) projection of the knee is taken for the demonstration of the
   A. tibial tuberosity
   B. condyles
   C. intercondyloid fossa
   D. patella

538. To what structure should the central ray be perpendicular when doing a tunnel view of the intercondyloid fossa?
   A. Popliteal depression
   B. Femoral condyles
   C. Tibial tuberosity
   D. Patellar apex

539. The true Holmblad view of the knee requires an angle of the tube of
   A. 0°
   B. 15° to 30°
   C. 35° to 45°
   D. 50° to 60°

540. The anteroposterior projection of the knee directs the central ray to the joint space with an angle of
   A. 0°
   B. 5° to 7° cephalad
   C. 10°
   D. 12° to 15° cephalad

541. Which structures function as shock absorbers for the knee?
   A. Bursae
   B. Menisci
   C. Ligaments
   D. Tendons

542. The projection usually utilized to demonstrate vertical fractures of the patella is the
    A. PA axial (Holmblad)
    B. tangential (Settegast)
    C. tangential (Kuchendorf)
    D. AP axial (Beclere)

543. The greater trochanter lies at the same level as which other palpable bony landmark?
    A. Symphysis pubis
    B. Coccyx
    C. Obturator foramen
    D. Anterior-superior iliac spine

544. When a patient is radiographed for a possible fracture of the hip, the radiographer positions the patient by the
    A. Freidman method
    B. Danelius-Miller method
    C. Johnson method
    D. Chassard-Lapine method

545. When radiographing the pelvis (AP), the femoral neck is BEST demonstrated by
    A. abducting the leg 30°
    B. inverting the feet 15°
    C. angling the tube 25° cephalad
    D. rotating the patient 45° oblique

546. Which of the following statements is INCORRECT?
    A. Scoliosis indicates a lateral curvature of the vertebrae
    B. Osteomalacia is an abnormal hardness of bones
    C. The epistropheus is found within the vertebrae
    D. The fabella is located in the region of the knee

547. Which of the following statements is **INCORRECT?**
- **A.** The AP projection of the ankle clearly demonstrates the upper portion of the astragalus
- **B.** The Alexander position is taken for the knee
- **C.** Osgood-Schlatters disease involves the tibial tuberosity
- **D.** Holmblad and Beclere are projections taken for the intercondyloid fossa

548. In order to position the pelvis properly in an AP position, the cassette should be centered to a point
- **A.** 2 in below the greater trochanter
- **B.** 2 in below the anterior superior iliac spine (ASIS)
- **C.** 2 in below the iliac crest
- **D.** 2 in below the ASIS

549. A true AP projection of the hip calls for a rotation of the foot approximately
- **A.** 10° eversion
- **B.** 15° inversion
- **C.** 20° abduction
- **D.** 35° extension

550. The crest of the ilium is at the same vertebral level as the
- **A.** first lumbar
- **B.** first and second sacrum
- **C.** eleventh thoracic
- **D.** fourth lumbar

551. The AP projection of the cervical spine demonstrates
- **A.** the atlas and axis
- **B.** the elongated spinous process
- **C.** all cervical vertebrae
- **D.** C3-T2

552. In order to project the atlas and axis, the central ray should be directed through the mouth at an angle that is

A. 15° caudad
B. 23° cephalad
C. parallel with the occlusal plane of the mandibular teeth
D. parallel with the occlusal plane of the maxillary teeth

553. Which of the following projections would **BEST** demonstrate the cervical intervertebral foramina?

A. PA oblique axial
B. Open mouth
C. Lateral
D. Extension

554. The intervertebral foramen contains the

1. blood vessels
2. spinal nerves
3. annulus fibrosus

A. 1 only
B. 1 and 2 only
C. 2 and 3 only
D. 1, 2, and 3

555. When radiographing the cervical spine AP, the lower anterior margins of the last four or five cervical vertebral bodies have a slightly lipped appearance which requires a(an)

A. 20° cephalad tube angulation
B. hyperextension
C. 30° flexion
D. 10° caudal tube angulation

556. Which of the following anatomical parts is **NOT** seen in the open mouth view?

A. Superior articular process
B. Transverse process
C. Body of C-1
D. Joint of Luschka

557. Which of the following is **NOT** clearly demonstrated in the lateral position of the thoracic spine?
  1. Pedicles
  2. Intervertebral foramina
  3. Intervertebral joint
  A. 1 only
  B. 2 only
  C. 1 and 2 only
  D. 1, 2, and 3

558. The technologist should be careful in collimating an AP dorsal spine projection that has been requested to rule out
  A. lordosis
  B. spina bifida
  C. kyphosis
  D. scoliosis

559. The (zygapophyseal) joints of the lumbar vertebra form an angle with the midsagittal plane of approximately
  A. 5° to 15°
  B. 20° to 30°
  C. 30° to 50°
  D. 50° to 60°

560. If a 10-in × 12-in cassette is used for the AP projection of the lumbar spine, the cassette is centered to a point
  A. 1 in superior to the iliac crest
  B. 2 to 3 in superior to the greater trochanter
  C. centered with the ASIS
  D. 3 in inferior from the umbilicus

561. Which statement is **INCORRECT**?
  A. The soft inner portion of the intervertebral disc is called the nucleus pulposus
  B. The dens epistropheal joint is located between C-1 and the occipital bone
  C. The roof of the orbits is formed by the frontal bone
  D. Most of the forehead is formed by the frontal bone

562. The normal L5-S1 junction forms an angle of
- **A.** 20° to 25°
- **B.** 30° to 35°
- **C.** 40° to 45°
- **D.** 60° to 80°

563. The intervertebral disks, which separate the individual vertebrae, are composed of
- **A.** elastic cartilage
- **B.** fibrocartilage
- **C.** hyaline cartilage
- **D.** osseous connective tissue

564. A lateral lumbar spine radiograph clearly demonstrates the
1. intervertebral foramen
2. spinous process
3. disk space
- **A.** 1 and 2 only
- **B.** 1 and 3 only
- **C.** 2 and 3 only
- **D.** 1, 2, and 3

565. In positioning the lumbar spine for a lateral view, with a 10-in × 12-in cassette, the technologist must direct the central ray 1.5 in superior to the level of the
- **A.** greater trochanter
- **B.** xiphoid process
- **C.** iliac crest
- **D.** symphysis pubis

566. In the AP projection of the sacrum, the tube is angled
- **A.** 10° caudad
- **B.** 15° cephalad
- **C.** 15° medially
- **D.** 45° caudad

567. Which of the following statements concerning anatomy of the chest is **CORRECT**?
   A. The esophagus is anterior to the trachea
   B. The right hilum is higher than the left hilum
   C. The diaphragm is higher posteriorly than anteriorly
   D. The right mainstem bronchus is shorter than the left mainstem bronchus

568. The anatomical landmark for localizing the bifurcation of the trachea into the mainstem bronchus is the
   A. xiphisternal joint
   B. sternal angle
   C. suprasternal notch
   D. tip of the xiphoid

569. Normally, a patient is asked to inhale deeply when having the lungs x-rayed. Which of the following is the **BEST** reason for that?
   A. More uniform density
   B. Increased contrast
   C. Greater magnification
   D. Greater area of lung structure shown

570. To demonstrate a pleural effusion in the chest of a patient who is unable to be put in an erect position, which of the following positions might you use?
   A. Transthoracic
   B. Supine
   C. Lateral decubitus
   D. Trendelenburg

571. Which of the following structures can be well-demonstrated on a lateral chest projection?
   A. Trachea
   B. Interlobar fissures
   C. Primary and secondary bronchi
   D. Mediastinum

572. Anterior oblique views of the chest demonstrate the
  1. heart
  2. aortic arch
  3. pulmonary artery
  A. 1 only
  B. 2 only
  C. 1 and 2 only
  D. 1, 2, and 3

573. When doing a PA chest to demonstrate the heart and aorta, the technologist should direct the central ray to
  A. T-1
  B. T-3
  C. T-5
  D. T-6

574. Which of the following structures is **NOT** well demonstrated on a lateral chest radiograph?
  A. Trachea
  B. Bronchi
  C. Heart
  D. Diaphragm

575. Which of the following oblique positions would require the greatest degree of rotation when performing a cardiac series?
  A. RPO
  B. LPO
  C. RAO
  D. LAO

576. The anteroposterior oblique position of the ribs requires the body to be rotated
  A. 20° to 30°, affected side toward the film
  B. 20° to 30°, affected side away from the film
  C. 45°, affected side toward the film
  D. 60°, affected side away from the film

577. The RPO position for radiography of the ribs will demonstrate an injury along the
    A. left margin
    B. costocartilage
    C. right margin
    D. facet

578. When radiographing the ribs below the diaphragm in the AP position, the central ray should be directed vertically to the level of
    A. T-6
    B. T-8
    C. T-12
    D. L-1

579. A posteroanterior axial projection of the clavicle requires a tube angulation of
    A. 10° to 15° caudad
    B. 15° to 20° cephalad
    C. 25° to 30° caudad
    D. 35° to 40° cephalad

580. A true lateral projection of the cranium will place the midsagittal plane
    A. perpendicular to the film
    B. parallel to the film
    C. 35° to the film
    D. 90° to the film

581. The mastoid tip is at the level of cervical vertebrae
    A. 1
    B. 2
    C. 3
    D. 4

582. The central ray for a PA projection of the cranium passes through the nasion at an angle of
A. 8° to 10° cephalad
B. 15° cephalad
C. 15° caudad
D. 25° caudad

583. For a reverse Towne position, the central ray enters the skull 1.5 in below the
A. mental point
B. external auditory meatus
C. external occipital protuberance
D. glabella

584. Which of the following projections would be **MOST** helpful in demonstrating a blow-out fracture?
A. Caldwell
B. Erect Waters
C. Basilar
D. Lateral facial

585. The **MOST** commonly fractured facial bone is the
A. nasal
B. mandible
C. maxillae
D. zygoma

586. The AP axial projection of the mandible is performed to demonstrate the
A. symphasis
B. raines
C. gonion
D. body

587. Which of the following projections will clearly demonstrate the crista galli?
   A. AP axial
   B. PA (Caldwell)
   C. Waters
   D. full basal

588. The Haas view will clearly demonstrate the
   1. dorsum sellae
   2. foramina ovale
   3. petrous pyramids
   A. 1 and 2 only
   B. 1 and 3 only
   C. 2 and 3 only
   D. 1, 2, and 3

589. The PA projection of the mandible **BEST** visualizes the
   A. mental foramina
   B. mandibular rami
   C. symphysis rami
   D. gonion

590. If a trauma patient is prone because of severe lacerations to the back, and the technologist is unable to obtain the routine Grashey position for the occipital, what method could be substituted?
   A. Caldwell
   B. Towne with a 60° angulation
   C. Rhese
   D. Haas

591. In a full basal projection of the skull, the infraorbitomeatal line should
   A. be as nearly parallel to the film as possible
   B. be perpendicular to the plane of the film
   C. form a 20° angle with the plane of the film
   D. form a 37° angle with the plane of the film

592. The cranial bone that is situated between the orbits and forms part of the anterior cranial fossa and part of the nasal and orbital walls is the
    A. ethmoid
    B. sphenoid
    C. frontal
    D. occipital

593. Which of the following bones does **NOT** help to form the bony orbit?
    A. Lacrimal
    B. Palatine
    C. Frontal
    D. Temporal

594. When performing a semiaxial skull, using the Townes method, which of the following items listed indicates proper angulation on the finished radiograph?
    A. Petrous ridges in lower third of orbits
    B. Dorsum sella in foramen magnum
    C. Petrous ridges projected inferior to the antra of Highmore
    D. Symmetry of orbital ridges

595. Located between the upper adjacent borders of the two parietal bones is a suture called the
    A. coronal
    B. squamosal
    C. sagittal
    D. lambdoidal

596. The slender, bony process extending forward from the temporal bone is the
    A. styloid
    B. zygomatic
    C. mastoid
    D. petrous

597. Which of the following is part of the mandible?
  1. Mental foramen
  2. Styloid process
  3. Coronoid process
    A. 1 and 2 only
    B. 1 and 3 only
    C. 2 and 3 only
    D. 1, 2, and 3

598. Which bone contains the semicircular canals?
    A. Occipital
    B. Sphenoid
    C. Ethmoid
    D. Temporal

599. Which statement is **INCORRECT**?
    A. The Caldwell projection demonstrates the frontal sinuses
    B. The Stenvers projection demonstrates the petrous ridges
    C. The Waters projection demonstrates the maxillary sinuses
    D. The Law projection demonstrates the optic foramina

600. Which of the following is the **MOST** superior sinus?
    A. Sphenoid
    B. Maxillary
    C. Frontal
    D. Ethmoid

601. Which of the following statements is **INCORRECT**?
    A. The clivus is located within the sphenoid
    B. The crista galli is located within the temporal
    C. The mastoid cells are found within the temporal
    D. The inion is located within the occipital

602. Which of the following bones is **NOT** considered part of the cranial floor?
    A. Frontal
    B. Sphenoid
    C. Ethmoid
    D. Temporal

603. One characteristic of the brachycephalic skull is that the petrous ridges form an angle with the midsagittal plane of
   A. 35°
   B. 47°
   C. 54°
   D. 60°

604. The Stenvers projection of the skull may be utilized for the demonstration of the
   A. internal auditory meatus
   B. maxillary sinuses
   C. zygomatic arch
   D. foramen magnum

605. Which of the following statements is **INCORRECT?**
   A. The floor of the skull is made up of six bones
   B. The vomer forms the lower part of the nasal septum
   C. The parietal forms the greater portion of the sides and roof of the cranium
   D. The pterygoids are found on the inferior surface of the sphenoid

606. The temporomandibular joint is formed by the mandibular fossa of the temporal bone and the
   A. ramus
   B. coracoid
   C. coronoid
   D. condyloid

607. In radiography of the nasal bones, the lateral projection will have the interpupillary line
   A. parallel to the TT
   B. perpendicular to the transorbital plane
   C. perpendicular to the TT
   D. parallel to the film

608. In order to position a patient properly for a reverse view of the optic foramen, you should adjust the head so that its medial sagittal plane will form with the plane of the film an angle of
  A. 53° with the acanthiomeatal line perpendicular
  B. 53° with the supraorbital line vertical
  C. 37° with the supraorbital line vertical
  D. 37° with the acanthiomeatal line vertical

609. The acanthiomeatal line is perpendicular to the film plane in a properly positioned
  A. Rhese
  B. Grashey
  C. Caldwell
  D. Arcelin

610. Skull sutures are classified as
  A. diarthroidal
  B. synarthroidal
  C. biarthroidal
  D. amphiarthroidal

611. The cochlea, housed within the petrous portion of the temporal bone, is concerned primarily with
  A. equilibrium
  B. sense of smell
  C. hearing
  D. balance

612. The thickest and densest part of the temporal bone is the portion termed the
  A. squamous
  B. petrous
  C. mastoid
  D. tympanic

613. In a routine Waters view for sinuses, the head is resting on the menti of the chin and the central ray is
- **A.** perpendicular to the film at the acanthion
- **B.** angled 15° cephalic to the nasion
- **C.** angled 20° to the glabella
- **D.** angled 35° caudad

614. A properly positioned Caldwell projection of the skull will demonstrate the
1. petrous pyramids
2. frontal sinuses
3. anterior ethmoid cells
- **A.** 1 and 2 only
- **B.** 1 and 3 only
- **C.** 2 and 3 only
- **D.** 1, 2, and 3

615. The Caldwell projection of the skull requires that the central ray be angled
- **A.** 15° to 20° caudad
- **B.** 25° to 35° caudad
- **C.** 15° cephalad
- **D.** 25° cephalad

616. Which projection demonstrates the dorsum sella and posterior clinoids projected through the foramen magnum of the skull?
- **A.** Anteroposterior
- **B.** Axial
- **C.** Submentovertical
- **D.** Lateral

617. The projection that is an exact reverse Stenvers is called a(an)
- **A.** Schuller's
- **B.** Law's
- **C.** Mayer's
- **D.** Arcelin's

618. The patient is prone, the midsagittal plane forms an angle of 45°
with the table top, and the infraorbitomeatal line is perpendicular to
the table top. This is called a
- **A.** Waters projection
- **B.** Stenvers projection
- **C.** Rhese projection
- **D.** Schuller projection

619. When positioning the sinuses in the Waters position, in order to
place the petrous portion of the temporal bones below the maxillary
antral floors, the
- **A.** orbitomeatal line forms an angle of 40° from the film plane
- **B.** midsagittal plane forms an angle of 37° from the film plane
- **C.** orbitomeatal line forms an angle of 37° from the film plane
- **D.** orbitomeatal line forms an angle of 53° from the film plane

620. The Stenvers position of the skull will demonstrate the
1. petrous ridge
2. mastoid antrum
3. internal auditory canal
- **A.** 1 and 2 only
- **B.** 1 and 3 only
- **C.** 2 and 3 only
- **D.** 1, 2, and 3

621. The subarachnoid space is located between the
- **A.** pia mater and arachnoid
- **B.** dura mater and arachnoid
- **C.** dura mater and pia mater
- **D.** dura mater and lamina

622. If a patient arrives in the emergency room on a spinal board for skull
and cervical spine radiographs, the radiographer's first exposure
would be taken in a
- **A.** flexion position
- **B.** cross-table lateral position
- **C.** oblique position
- **D.** open-mouth position

623. Which of the following bones contains a paranasal sinus?
   A. Temporal
   B. Sphenoid
   C. Parietal
   D. Occipital

624. A slightly movable joint is classified as being
   A. synarthrodial
   B. amphiarthrodial
   C. diarthrodial
   D. semiarthrodial

625. The articulations of the mandible are an example of which type of joint?
   A. Diarthrodial
   B. Amphiarthrodial
   C. Synathrodial
   D. Transarthrodial

626. Blood is transported via the four pulmonary veins to the
   A. left ventricle
   B. aorta
   C. superior vena cava
   D. left atrium

627. Blood flowing away from the heart passes through the abdominal aorta and then into the
   A. left and right common iliac artery
   B. right and left femorals
   C. left and right common carotids
   D. right and left celiacs

628. Which of the following blood vessels connect to the liver?
    1. Inferior vena cava
    2. Hepatic artery
    3. Hepatic portal vein
  A. 1 and 2 only
  B. 1 and 3 only
  C. 2 and 3 only
  D. 1, 2, and 3

629. The abdominal aorta bifurcates into the right and left
  A. subclavian arteries
  B. axillary arteries
  C. common iliac arteries
  D. popliteal arteries

630. The right and left brachiocephalic veins join to form the
  A. cephalic vein
  B. jugular vein
  C. inferior vena cava
  D. superior vena cava

631. The cerebral artery that appears closest to midline on an AP or Towne projection during an angiogram is the
  A. anterior cerebral
  B. middle cerebral
  C. posterior cerebral
  D. carotid siphon

632. The innominate artery will branch into the
  A. left and right common carotid
  B. left subclavian and right subclavian
  C. right common carotid and right vertebral
  D. right common carotid and right subclavian

633. The trachea bifurcates at the level of
  A. C-7
  B. D-2
  C. D-5
  D. D-8

634. The vessel that carries blood from the right ventricle to the lungs is the
- **A.** aorta
- **B.** pulmonary artery
- **C.** subclavian artery
- **D.** superior vena cava

635. The common bile duct is formed by the junction of the cystic duct and the
- **A.** common hepatic duct
- **B.** cystic duct
- **C.** sphincter of Oddi
- **D.** fundus of gallbladder

636. The curved portion of the colon between the rectum and descending colon is the
- **A.** cecum
- **B.** sigmoid
- **C.** left colic flexure
- **D.** appendix

637. A properly exposed scout abdomen radiograph should demonstrate the
1. psoas muscles
2. kidneys
3. inferior margin of the liver
- **A.** 1 and 2 only
- **B.** 1 and 3 only
- **C.** 2 and 3 only
- **D.** 1, 2, and 3

638. The barium enema is contraindicated if the physician suspects
- **A.** ileus
- **B.** diverticulitis
- **C.** acute appendicitis
- **D.** stricture

639. In order to place the kidneys parallel to the film when doing right and left obliques, the technologist should turn the patient approximately
   A. 10°
   B. 20°
   C. 30°
   D. 45°

640. Ureteric compression should **NOT** be performed on patients suffering from
   1. possible ureteral calculi
   2. abdominal mass
   3. aortic aneurysm
   A. 1 and 2 only
   B. 1 and 3 only
   C. 2 and 3 only
   D. 1, 2, and 3

641. A toxic condition associated with renal insufficiency and retention in the blood of nitrogeneous substances normally excreted by the kidneys is known as
   A. uremia
   B. anemia
   C. dysuria
   D. urethritis

642. Which of the following procedures is considered a nonfunctional study?
   1. Retrograde urography
   2. Excretory urography
   3. Hypertensive excretory urography
   A. 1 only
   B. 1 and 2 only
   C. 2 and 3 only
   D. 1, 2, and 3

643. Compression is used during excretory urography in order to accomplish which one of the following?
A. Aiding in the excretion process
B. Immobilizing the patient
C. Preventing the patient from breathing during the exposure
D. Retaining the contrast medium in the collecting system

644. An obstruction in the common bile duct before surgery is demonstrated by the following radiographic procedures(s).
1. Percutaneous transhepatic cholangiography
2. T-tube cholangiography
3. Intravenous cholangiography
A. 1 and 2 only
B. 1 and 3 only
C. 2 and 3 only
D. 1, 2, and 3

645. Ova travels from the ovaries to the uterus by way of the
A. alimentary canal
B. eustachian tubes
C. fallopian tubes
D. seminal duct

646. The part of the brain that controls cardiac function and respiration is termed the
A. pons
B. medulla oblongata
C. hypothalamus
D. cerebellum

647. Which of the following is a radiographic study of the urinary bladder that involves the direct injection of a contrast media through a catheter?
A. Intravenous pyelogram
B. Intravenous urogram
C. Retrograde pyelogram
D. Cystogram

648. Which of the following is a cholecystagogic?
   A. Renografin
   B. Cholex or Neo-Cholex
   C. Con-Ray
   D. Hypaque

649. Which of the following procedures is commonly performed on a nongravid patient?
   1. Aminography
   2. Pelvic pneumograph
   3. Hysterosalpingography
   A. 1 and 2 only
   B. 1 and 3 only
   C. 2 and 3 only
   D. 1, 2, and 3

650. Hysterosalpingography is performed to evaluate the
   1. tubal passages
   2. size and shape of the pubic arch
   3. uterine cavity
   A. 1 and 2 only
   B. 1 and 3 only
   C. 2 and 3 only
   D. 1, 2, and 3

651. Cholecystocholangiography is performed to demonstrate the
   A. kidneys, uterus, and bladder
   B. gallbladder and bile ducts
   C. splenic and hepatic flexures
   D. stomach and small intestine

652. If a scout film of the abdomen taken for an oral cholecystogram demonstrates numerous radiopaque stones, the radiographer should
   A. continue with the additional films
   B. withhold the stimulant and bring the film to the attention of the radiologist
   C. give the patient a gallbladder stimulant and take an erect film in one-half hour
   D. take three oblique views of the patient at 15° intervals

653. Pancreatic enzymes travel along the pancreatic duct and empty into the
   A. duodenum
   B. ileum
   C. jejunum
   D. liver

654. Which of the following positions would be **LEAST** useful when radiographing a very thin patient for a gallbladder series?
   A. AP
   B. LAO
   C. RPO
   D. Right lateral decubitus

655. Which of the following areas would **NOT** be demonstrated on an IVC?
   A. Common bile duct
   B. Glomerular duct
   C. Hepatic duct
   D. Cystic duct

656. To demonstrate the stratification of cholecystoliths, the patient is placed in
   A. left lateral decubitus
   B. Fowler position
   C. right lateral decubitus
   D. left posterior oblique

657. The cystic duct from the gallbladder empties into which of the following?
   A. Right hepatic duct
   B. Common bile duct
   C. Left hepatic duct
   D. Duct of Wirsung

658. The right posterior oblique (RPO) and left posterior oblique (LPO) projections for a barium enema are used to demonstrate the
A. sigmoid
B. right and left colic flexures
C. ileo-cecal junction
D. recto-sigmoid junction

659. During oral cholecystography, which position will **BEST** demonstrate the cystic duct and common bile duct after the patient has ingested a cholecystogogue?
A. AP erect
B. RPO 15° to 30°
C. LAO 15° to 30°
D. Right lateral decubitus

660. In order to keep the contrast agent in the kidneys for a long period of time, the technologist may
 1. apply ureteric compression
 2. tilt the table 15° (Trendelenburg)
 3. do a 20-minute LPO 30° erect film
A. 1 and 2 only
B. 1 and 3 only
C. 2 and 3 only
D. 1, 2, and 3

661. Which of the following is **NOT** seen on an IVP radiograph five minutes after injection?
A. Renal pyramid
B. Calyx (major and minor)
C. Renal pelvis
D. Urethra

662. A patient who has a stomach and gallbladder in a higher than normal position would be referred to as being
A. hypersthenic
B. sthenic
C. hyposthenic
D. asthenic

663. During an IVC, the time after injection for optimal visualization of
the bile ducts is usually about
A. 10 to 20 minutes
B. 25 to 35 minutes
C. 40 to 80 minutes
D. 1.5 to 2 hours

664. The gallbaldder is well visualized by the use of
A. cholecystokinin
B. cholecystogogue
C. cholecystoliths
D. cholecystopaques

665. Large tortuous veins of the esophagus are known as
A. tracheal-esophageal varices
B. esophageal varicies
C. hemorrhoids
D. tracheal varicies

666. In which of the following positions would the stomach be **MOST**
superior?
A. Right lateral with inspiration
B. Erect with inspiration
C. Left posterior oblique with expiration
D. Right anterior oblique with expiration

667. In reference to the stomach, which of the following **BEST** describes
the location of the fundus in relation to the pylorus?
1. Anterior
2. Posterior
3. Superior
A. 1 and 2 only
B. 1 and 3 only
C. 2 and 3 only
D. 1, 2, and 3

668. Which portion of the small intestine is the longest?
- **A.** Jejunum
- **B.** Pylorus
- **C.** Duodenum
- **D.** Ileum

669. When performing a barium enema, the hepatic flexure can **BEST** be demonstrated by placing the patient
- **A.** AP axial
- **B.** left AP oblique
- **C.** left PA oblique
- **D.** right AP oblique

670. Right anterior oblique radiographs of the stomach filled with $BaSO_4$ and a high kilovoltage technique will usually demonstrate the
- **A.** duodenal bulb
- **B.** distal esophagus
- **C.** greater curvature
- **D.** upper stomach

671. Most gastric ulcers appear within the
- **A.** duodenum
- **B.** greater curvature of the stomach
- **C.** fundus
- **D.** lesser curve of the stomach

672. The opening located between the esophagus and the stomach is called the
- **A.** pyloric antrum
- **B.** cardiac orifice
- **C.** duodenum
- **D.** pyloric orifice

673. During a GI series, the Trendeleburg position is sometimes utilized in order to demonstrate a(an)
- **A.** esophageal reflux
- **B.** hiatal hernia
- **C.** duodenal lesions
- **D.** gastric ulcers

674. During an upper GI, a retrogastric mass can be demonstrated when the patient is positioned in a
  A. lateral position
  B. erect position
  C. left posterior oblique position
  D. prone position

675. The position of the stomach that demonstrates barium in the pyloric antrum and air in the fundus is the
  A. LPO
  B. LAO
  C. AP
  D. PA

676. In the left lateral decubitus, air will form shadows under the
  A. spleen
  B. stomach
  C. pancreas
  D. right hemidiaphragm

677. The patient position that will clearly demonstrate the barium-filled pyloric canal and duodenum is the
  A. Fowler
  B. RAO
  C. AP
  D. LPO

678. The normal position for the ureters' entrance to the urinary bladder is
  A. superior medial
  B. anterior lateral
  C. inferior medial
  D. posterior lateral

679. The proximal expanded tip of the ureter at the union of the major calyces is called the renal
    A. capsule
    B. pelvis
    C. cortex
    D. pyramid

680. The usual dose of contrast media for adults having an IVP is approximately
    A. 10 to 20 mL
    B. 30 to 100 mL
    C. 100 to 150 mL
    D. 150 to 200 mL

681. In the urinary system, the collecting tubules and loop of Henle are located in the
    A. cortex
    B. medulla
    C. hilus
    D. calyces

682. The basic position utilized for a male patient having a voiding cystourethrogram is the
    A. AP
    B. LAO
    C. RPO
    D. PA

683. One of the procedures used to investigate the blood vessels of the liver and spleen is the
    A. abdominal aortogram
    B. femoral arteriogram
    C. lymphangiogram
    D. percutaneous cholangiogram

684. Endoscopic retrograde cholangiopancreatography (ERCP) is performed to evaluate the
  A. liver
  B. biliary system
  C. duodenum
  D. colon

685. Which of the following procedures would **MOST** likely follow an excretory urogram?
  A. Cholangiography
  B. Proctology
  C. Retrograde pyelography
  D. Amniography

686. Which of the following substances would **NOT** be used in an oral cholecystogram?
  A. Oragrafin
  B. Cholografin
  C. Neo-Cholex
  D. Telepaque

687. Gallstones are usually composed of
  1. cholesterol
  2. bile pigment
  3. calcium salts
  A. 1 only
  B. 1 and 2 only
  C. 2 and 3 only
  D. 1, 2, and 3

688. Which of the following radiographic procedures should **ALWAYS** be performed with a strict aseptic technique?
  A. Oral cholecystography
  B. Voiding cystography
  C. Angiography
  D. Body section radiography

689. Which of the following should be used in order to ensure an acceptable amount of image sharpness during mammography?
A. Air gap technique
B. Fractional focal spot
C. Subtraction technique
D. High-speed screens

690. The hormone that stimulates the liver to convert glycogen to glucose is
A. ADH
B. cortisol
C. glucagon
D. insulin

691. Which of the following conditions is unrelated to the small intestine?
A. Meckel's diverticulum
B. leiomyomas
C. Crohn's disease
D. Hirschsprung's disease

692. A patient complaining of persistent cyanosis and edema in one or both legs would probably have which of the following exams done?
A. Myelogram
B. Aortogram
C. Lymphangiogram
D. Venogram

693. Which of the following views for mammography would demonstrate the **MOST** tissue of the breast?
A. Anterior
B. Mediolateral
C. Axillary
D. AP

694. Arthrography films should clearly demonstrate the
1. menisci and bursae
2. ligaments
3. articular cartilage
   A. 1 only
   B. 1 and 2 only
   C. 2 and 3 only
   D. 1, 2, and 3

695. When translumbar aortography is performed, the contrast media is injected into the
   A. groin and allowed to ascend to the heart
   B. groin with a pressure injector
   C. foot and allowed to ascend to the heart
   D. abdominal aorta

696. When performing lymphadenography, how long after the injection is the examination made?
   A. One hour
   B. Three hours
   C. 12 hours
   D. 24 hours

697. Which of the following examinations is **BEST** made within the 40 to 55 kV range?
   A. Myelography
   B. Xeromammography
   C. Pneumoencephalography
   D. Kymomgraphy

698. The puncture site for a lumbar myelogram is usually between
   A. D-12 and L-1
   B. L-1 and L-2
   C. L-2 and L-4
   D. L-5 and S-1

699. When performing abdominal aortography, the central ray is directed to the level of
   A. D-12
   B. L-2
   C. L-4
   D. S-1

700. The puncture site for myelography is performed at the vertebral interspace of L-3 and L-4 because
   A. the interspace is wider
   B. the cord is not present
   C. less nerve roots are present
   D. the spinal canal is wider

Explanatory Answers

451. A.   When positioning the cranium for the posteroanterior projection, the orbitomeatal line is perpendicular to the table. (Ref. 5, p. 213)

452. B.   The parasagittal and sagittal planes do not pass through the midline, but divide the body into right and left portions. The coronal plane divides the body into anterior and posterior portions. (Ref. 37, p. 11)

453. A.   The epigastrium or epigastric region is located "upon the stomach," superior to the umbilical region. (Ref. 37, p. 17)

454. D.   Abduction refers to a movement of the arm or leg away from the body, a lateral movement (draw away from). (Ref. 5, p. 30)

455. A.   Eversion is an outward movement of the foot at the ankle joint. (Ref. 5, p. 29)

456. D.   The junctions of the upper and lower eyelids are termed canthi. (Ref. 5, p. 203)

457. C.   The glabella is a smooth prominence between the eyebrows and above the bridge of the nose. (Ref. 5, p. 202)

458. A.   The ventral body cavity has two principal subdivisions, the (upper) thoracic and the (lower) abdominopelvic cavity. (Ref. 37, p. 12)

459. C.   The body of the stomach is located in the left upper quadrant. (Ref. 37, p. 19)

460. A.   The duodenum is located in the right upper quadrant.(Ref. 37, p. 19)

461. C.   The urinary bladder is located in the (pubic) hypogastric region. (Ref. 27. p. 17)

462. B.   The gallbladder is located below the liver in the right hypochondriac region. (Ref. 37, p. 17)

463. A. The gallbladder is anterior to the hepatic and bile ducts. (Ref. 5, p. 426)

464. B. The xiphisternal joint is located at the level of the ninth thoracic vertebra. (Ref. 32, p. 147)

465. C. 22 cm + 34 cm = 56 cm ÷ 2 = 28 cm.(Ref. 5, p. 49)

466. C. The kidneys are usually located at the level of T-12 to L-3 vertebra. (Ref. 5, p. 445)

467. B. The hypersthenic body type designates the massive body build. (Ref. 5, p. 362)

468. B. The average body build is the sthenic type. (Ref. 5, p. 362)

469. B. Legg-Calvé Perthes disease is a osteochondritis of the upper femoral epiphysis. (Ref. 34, p. 1011)

470. B. The gallbladder is higher and more to the right in the hypersthenic body type than in the sthenic type. (Ref. 5, p. 362)

471. B. Dysplastic tissue displays a highly abnormal, but not clearly cancerous, appearance. (Ref. 1, p. 299)

472. A. Ewing's tumor or sarcoma is a diffuse endothelioma or endothelial myeloma forming a fusiform swelling on a long bone. (Ref. 34, p. 631)

473. B. Agenesis is the failure of an organ or part to develop or grow. (Ref. 34, p. 50)

474. C. Metastasis is the process by which tumor cells are spread to distance parts of the body. (Ref. 1, p. 561)

475. C. Impaction relates to a fractured bone that is mashed together. (Ref. 34, p. 897)

476. B. Hodgkin's disease is a malignant condition causing enlargement of lymphoid tissue, spleen, liver, and other tissues. (Ref. 34, p. 836)

477. A. Osteoporosis is a disorder characterized by abnormal rarefaction of bone, occurring most frequently in postmenopausal women. (Ref. 1, p. 643)

478. B. A Colle's fracture occurs at the distal end of the radius. (Ref. 34, p. 383)

479. C. The prefix *para* relates to near or beside. (Ref. 23, p. 64)

480. B. Apoplexy is a cerebrovascular accident resulting in paralysis. (Ref. 17, p. 87)

481. D. An avulsion is a tearing away forcibly of a part or a structure of tendinous attachment to the osseous tissue. (Ref. 34, p. 173)

482. B. The term osteomyelitis includes all infectious diseases of bone involving periosteum, marrow, and cartilage. (Ref. 17, p. 583)

483. A. Osteomalacia is a demineralization or "softening" of the bones of the pelvis, legs, and spine from a vitamin D deficiency. (Ref. 17, p. 583)

484. C. A tripod fracture occurs at the zygoma at its three sutures: frontal, temporal, and maxillary. The other types occur in the foot. (Ref. 24, p. 268)

485. D. An osteochondroma is a benign tumor made of bone and cartilage. (Ref. 17, p. 852)

486. A. Atherosclerosis is a common arterial disorder characterized by yellowish plaques of cholesterol, lipids, and cellular debris in the walls of large- and medium-sized arteries. (Ref. 17, p. 106)

487. D. An idiopathic disease is one that arises without an apparent cause. (Ref. 17, p. 602)

488. A. A spontaneous or neoplastic fracture results from weakened bone tissue caused by a neoplasm or by a malignant growth. (Ref. 17, p. 801)

489. B. Arthography can involve the injection of both a negative and a positive contrast medium. (Ref. 5, p. 563)

490. D. The newest method for myelography involves an aqueous contrast medium of metrizamide, called Amipaque. (Ref. 13, p. 195)

491. B. Barium sulfate is an inert organic salt of the chemical element barium. It forms a suspension when mixed with water. (Ref. 13, p. 176)

492. C. Ethiodol or ethiodized oil has approved usage for lymphography. (Ref. 13, p. 192)

493. B. A flush feeling in the face and a metallic taste are two common side effects following contrast media injection. (Ref. 5, p. 450)

494. B. The urologist injects 3 to 5 cc of any of the urographic contrast medias directly into the renal pelvis of one or both kidneys. (Ref. 5, p. 457)

495. A. In general, approximately 4 mL are required to fill a normal uterine cavity. An additional 4 mg may be required to visualize the fallopian tubes. (Ref. 30, p. 189)

496. B. Pneumoarthrography uses air or other easily absorbed gases. (Ref. 30, p. 196)

497. D. Cholografin meglumine is the approved contrast medium for IV cholangiography. (Ref. 13, p. 194)

498. B. Meglumine contrast agents are used mainly for urographic studies under the brand names of Bilopaque, Cholebrine, Oragrafil (calcium or sodium), and Telepaque. (Ref. 13, p. 194)

499. B. The lymph vessel and lymph nodes are demonstrated by direct injection of ethiodol. (Ref. 13, p. 195)

500. B. The Danielus-Miller position is utilized during surgical hip procedures. (Ref. 5, p. 192)

501. B. To reduce the possibility of blood clot formation, catheter and guidewire manufacturers have designed their products to be coated with heparin. (Ref. 38, p. 149)

502. D. The trapezium is the first of the carpals in the distal row from the lateral to medial position articulating with the first metacarpal. (Ref. 3, p. 52)

503. A. Separate positioning prevents rotation distortion because of central ray location; however, if you wish to limit exposure to a young patient, you may expose both hands with one exposure. (Ref. 3, p. 73)

504. B. The pisiform and hamate are best visualized in the carpal canal position. (Ref. 5, p. 88)

505. A. The three carpals involved in the wrist joint are the scaphoid, lunate, and triangular. (Ref. 5, p. 89)

506. B. The only carpal that articulates with the first metacarpal is the greater multangular. (Ref. 5, p. 87)

507. D. For a lateral elbow, it should be flexed 90° with the humerus and forearm in contact with the table. (Ref. 3, p. 92)

508. A. The medial oblique projection of the elbow shows the coronoid process free of superimposition. (Ref. 3, p. 94)

509. B. The "fat pad" is a small accumulation of fat adjacent to the anterior surface of the distal humerus, as demonstrated in the lateral position. (Ref. 24, p. 40)

510. B. Just below the head of the humerus, lying on the same oblique plane, is the narrow constricted anatomic neck. (Ref. 5, p. 114)

511. B. The most proximal end of the ulna contains the olecranon process, which forms the prominence of the elbow. (Ref. 3, p. 53)

512. C. The trochlea of the distal humerus articulates with the semilunar notch of the ulna to form the hinge joint of the elbow. (Ref. 3, p. 53)

513. A. The acromion is formed by the end of the spine of the scapula and is a flattened, expanded process. (Ref. 37, p. 191)

514. D. The bicipital groove, or intertubercular sulcus, is a prominent depression of the proximal humerus located between the greater and lesser tubercles. (Ref. 37, p. 191)

515. D. The articular portion of the humeral condyle on the medial side is the trochlea. The capitellum is on the lateral side. (Ref. 5, p. 106)

516. D. The greater tuberosity is best demonstrated by external rotation. (Ref. 5, p. 118)

517. A. The central ray should be centered to the coracoid process for anteroposterior projection of the shoulder. (Ref. 5, p. 128)

518. B. The transaxillar lateral position is for nontrauma cases. (Ref. 5, p. 129)

519. D. The glenoid fossa is the thickest part of the scapula and ends in a shallow depression. (Ref. 5, p. 123)

520. D. The transthoracic lateral position clearly demonstrates the proximal humerus and the relationship of the glenohumeral joint. (Ref. 5, p. 132)

521. B. The AP, internal, and external rotation projections are used to demonstrate possible calcium deposits in muscles, tendons, or bursar structures of the shoulder. (Ref. 5, p. 127)

522. A. The coracoid process projects off the anterior scapula; the coronoid process is on the proximal ulna. (Ref. 37, p. 193)

523. C. The medial oblique shows the interspace between the cuboid and fourth and fifth metatarsals. (Ref. 3, p. 178)

194 / Radiography

524. B. The dorsoplantar projection of the foot requires a 10° angle toward the heel. (Ref. 5, p. 177)

525. A. The scaphoid (navicular) lies on the medial side of the foot, between the talus and the three cuneiforms. (Ref. 5, p. 163)

526. C. The plantodorsal projection of the calcaneus has the central ray form an angle of 40° with the long axis of the foot. (Ref. 3, p. 193)

527. D. The medial oblique position shows the tarsals free of superimposition. (Ref. 5, p. 152)

528. D. In the medial oblique position, the foot is rotated medially 45°. (Ref. 5, p. 152)

529. B. The AP ankle demonstrates the distal tibia and fibula, talus, and ankle joint. (Ref. 5, p. 156)

530. D. The AP ankle clearly demonstrates the upper portion of astragalus (talus). (Ref. 3, p. 204)

531. B. The lateral malleolus is particularly well shown in the medial oblique projection. (Ref. 3, p. 207)

532. D. To ensure that the leg is in a true lateral position, palpation of the malleoli and epicondyles is critical. (Ref. 5, p. 169)

533. B. The anteriomedial oblique projection separates the proximal ends of the tibia and fibula. (Ref. 3, p. 221)

534. D. The anatomical position places the first metatarsal proximal; therefore, the third metatarsal would be lateral to the second metatarsal. (Ref. 5, p. 141)

535. B. To demonstrate the patella in the lateral position, you would flex the leg no more than 5°. (Ref. 5, p. 174)

536. B. To properly center the knee joint, the central ray is directed to a point 1 cm inferior to the apex of the patella. (Ref. 5, p. 170)

537. C. The semiaxial PA projection, or tunnel position, will clearly demonstrate the intercondyloid fossa, distal femur, tibial spine, tibial plateau, and knee joint. (Ref. 5, p. 176)

538. A. The tube is angled 40° to the popliteal depression when demonstrating the intercondyloid fossa. (Ref. 3, p. 226)

539. A. The true Holmblad upright, standing, or kneeling requires a vertical 0° beam. (Ref. 3, p. 224)

540. B. The AP knee projection requires a 5° to 7° cephalad angle of the tube. (Ref. 5, p. 170)

541. B. The menisci are sometimes called "shock absorbers" of the knee. (Ref. 5, p. 164)

542. B. The Settegest projection is used to demonstrate vertical fractures of the patella. (Ref. 3, p. 235)

543. A. The most prominent point of the greater trochanter is in the same transverse plane as the symphysis pubis. (Ref. 3, p. 245)

544. B. The axiolateral (Danelius-Miller) projection is used in trauma hip cases. (Ref. 3, p. 260)

545. B. A 15° internal rotation of the feet will overcome the anteversion of the femoral necks and place their long axes parallel with the plane of the film. (Ref. 3, p. 246)

546. B. Osteosclerosis is an abnormal hardness of bones. (Ref. 17, p. 854)

547. B. The Alexander method is used for acromioclavicular articulations and optic foramen studies. (Ref. 3, p. 140)

548. B. For the AP pelvis projection, the central ray is directed to a point midway between the symphysis pubis and iliac crest. (Ref. 3, p. 246)

196 / Radiography

549. B. A 15° to 20° inversion of the affected leg overcomes the anteversion present. (Ref. 3, p. 256)

550. D. The iliac crest is at the same level as L-4. (Ref. 32, p. 147)

551. D. The anteroposterior projection of the cervical vertebrae with a 15° tube angulation shows C3-C7. (Ref. 3, p. 301)

552. D. The head should be adjusted so that a line from the lower edge of the upper incisors to the tip of the mastoid process is perpendicular to the film, with the central ray directed perpendicular. (Ref. 3, p. 292)

553. A. Anterior obliques of the cervical spine demonstrate the intervertebral foramina and pedicles closest to the film. (Ref. 3, p. 309)

554. B. The intervertebral foramina contain the spinal nerves and blood vessels. (Ref. 3, p. 281)

555. A. For the lower cervical vertebra, the central ray is angled 20° cephalad at the level of the thyroid cartilage. (Ref. 3, p. 301)

556. D. The odontoid view shows C-1 and C-2, the lateral masses, and the occipital base. (Ref. 3, p. 293)

557. A. The pedicles are not demonstrated by the lateral position, but are clearly seen in the anteroposterior projection. (Ref. 3, p. 323)

558. D. With the x-ray beam collimated inside the breast shadows, severe scoliosis cases could extend out of the field. (Ref. 3, p. 358)

559. C. The normal angle of the apophysial joints of the lumbar vertebra is 30° to 50°. (Ref. 3, p. 287)

560. A. The central ray entering approximately 1 in superior to the iliac crest will place it on L-3. (Ref. 3, p. 331)

561. B. The dens epistropheal joint is found between C-1 and C-2. (Ref. 3, p. 294)

562. B. The normal angle between L5-S1 is approximately 30° to 35°. (Ref. 5, p. 295)

563. B. Fibrocartilage is found in the symphasis pubis and forms the disks between the vertebrae. (Ref. 3, p. 281)

564. D. The lateral lumbar spinous process will clearly demonstrate the intervertebral disk space, intervertebral foramina, and the spinous process. (Ref. 3, p. 337)

565. C. In order to direct the central ray to L-3, center 1 to 1.5 in above the top of the iliac crest. (Ref. 3, p. 336)

566. B. To clearly demonstrate the sacrum in the AP projection requires a 15° cephalad tube angulation. (Ref. 3, p. 350)

567. D. The right bronchus has a shorter distance to reach the individual lobes. (Ref. 5, p. 40)

568. B. The sternal angle corresponds to the second rib and T-5, where the bifurcation of the trachea exists. (Ref. 5, p. 39)

569. D. Full inspiration on a chest radiograph will demonstrate maximum lung structures. (Ref. 5, p. 49)

570. C. The lateral decubitus positions of the chest demonstrate air-fluid levels in the pleural space. (Ref. 5, p. 56)

571. B. The lateral chest position demonstrates interlobar fissures and pulmonary lesions. (Ref. 3, p. 415)

572. D. Right anterior oblique and left anterior oblique chest projections demonstrate the heart, descending aorta, and pulmonary artery. (Ref. 3, p. 416)

573. D. In the PA projection, the central ray is directed to the level of the sixth dorsal vertebra. (Ref. 5, p. 49)

574. B. The lateral chest position demonstrates lungs, trachea, heart and great vessels, and diaphragm. (Ref. 5, p. 51)

575. D. When performing a cardiac series, the RAO is taken at 40° and the LAO is taken at 60°. (Ref. 5, p. 372)

576. C. For posterior oblique projections of the ribs, the side of injury is closest to the film. (Ref. 5, p. 340)

577. C. Anterior oblique projections of the ribs demonstrate the axillary borders. (Ref. 5, p. 340)

578. C. The central ray is directed perpendicular to the film holder at T-12 to best show the lower pairs of ribs. (Ref. 5, p. 339)

579. A. The PA axial projection of the clavicle requires a tube angle of 10° to 15° caudad. (Ref. 5, p. 133)

580. B. In a lateral position of the cranium, the midsagittal plane is parallel to the table or film. (Ref. 5, p. 212)

581. A. The mastoid tip is found at the level of the atlas or C-1. (Ref. 3, p. 38)

582. C. In the PA projection of the cranium, the central ray passes through the nasion with a 15° caudad angle. (Ref. 5, p. 213)

583. C. In the PA axial (Haas) projection of the cranium, the central ray enters 1.5 in below the inion, and emerges 1 in above the nasion. (Ref. 3, p. 237)

584. B. The erect Waters can demonstrate an air level seen in the upper orbit when the orbital floor is fractured. (Ref. 5, p. 232)

585. A. The most commonly fractured facial bone is the nasal bone. It may be accompanied by a fracture of the ascending process of the maxillae and/or nasal septum. (Ref. 24, p. 57)

586. B.   The AP axial (intraoral) position is an oblique occlusal position of the region of the mandibular symphasis. (Ref. 3, p. 331)

587. B.   The PA (Caldwell) will clearly demonstrate the frontal bone, greater and lesser wings, crista galli, petrous ridges, and internal auditory canal. (Ref. 5, p. 213)

588. B.   The foramina ovale are not demonstrated on a Haas projection. (Ref. 3, p. 237)

589. B.   The PA mandible shows either mandibular body or the rami and temporomandibular joints. (Ref. 3, p. 336)

590. D.   The Haas method demonstrates a symmetric view of the petrous pyramids and dorsum sellae within the shadow of the foramen magnum. (Ref. 3, p. 237)

591. A.   In the SMV projection of the skull, the infraorbitomeatal line should be parallel with the film. (Ref. 5, p. 215)

592. A.   The ethmoid bone is a small, cube-shaped bone. It helps form the anterior cranial fossa and part of the nasal and orbital walls. (Ref. 5, p. 209)

593. D.   The bony orbit is formed by seven bones: sphenoid, ethmoid, lacrimal, maxillae, palatine, zygoma, and frontal. (Ref. 3, p. 256)

594. B.   In a well-positioned occipital or Towne position of the skull, the dorsum sellae is clearly projected into the foramen magnum. (Ref. 5, p. 214)

595. C.   The sagittal suture is one of the four prominent skull sutures located between the two parietal bones. (Ref. 5, p. 206)

596. A.   The styloid process projects downward from the undersurface of the temporal bone and serves as a point of attachment for muscles and ligaments of the tongue and neck. (Ref. 5, p. 207)

597. B.   The coronoid process is the point on the mandible where the temporalis muscles attach. The mental foramen is an opening where the mental nerve and vessels pass. (Ref. 5, p. 246)

598. D. The semicircular canals consist of an anterior, posterior, and lateral semicircular canal, and are found within the vestibulocochleal organ of the temporal bone. (Ref. 3, p. 213)

599. D. The Law projection demonstrates the mastoid processes. (Ref. 3, p. 390)

600. C. The frontal sinuses are located between the inner and outer tables of the skull, posterior to the glabella. (Ref. 5, p. 248)

601. B. The crista galli is part of the ethmoid. (Ref. 5, p. 209)

602. A. The cranial floor is made up of the sphenoid, ethmoid, and the right and left temporal bones. The frontal bone is found in the calvarium, or skull cap. (Ref. 5, p. 205)

603. C. An angle greater than 40° (approximately 54°) is found in the brachycephalic skull. (Ref. 5, p. 210)

604. A. The Stenvers position demonstrates the mastoid process, petrous ridge, tympanic cavity, bony labyrinth, and internal auditory meatus. (Ref. 5, p. 270)

605. A. The floor of the skull is made up of four bones. They are sphenoid, ethmoid, and right and left temporals. (Ref. 5, p. 205)

606. D. The condyle of the condyloid process fits into the temporomandibular fossa of the temporal bone to form the temporomandibular joint (tmj). (Ref. 5, p. 245)

607. C. The interpupillary line is perpendicular to the film for the lateral position of nasal bones. (Ref. 5, p. 236)

608. A. The orbitoparietal oblique projection requires a 53° rotation of the head. (Ref. 3, p. 260)

609. A. In positioning the patient for a Rhese position, adjust the flexion of the head to place the acanthiomeatal line perpendicular to the plane of the film. (Ref. 3, p. 258)

610. B. The articulations or joints of the skull called sutures belong in the synarthrodial or immovable category. (Ref. 5, p. 206)

611. C. The vestibulococlear organ, or organ of hearing, contains the cochlea. (Ref. 3, p. 213)

612. B. The petrous pyramid, or pars petrosa, is the pyramid-shaped portion of the temporal bone and is the thickest and densest bone in the cranium. (Ref. 5, p. 207)

613. A. In the Waters view for sinuses, the central ray enters the posterior sagittal suture and exits at the acanthion. (Ref. 5, p. 263)

614. C. The Caldwell position will also demonstrate the crista galli and internal auditory canals. (Ref. 5, p. 213)

615. A. The Caldwell projection for the cranium employs a 15° caudad tube angulation. (Ref. 5, p. 213)

616. B. In the axial projection, the occipital region is free of superimposition and allows for demonstration of the dorsum sellae and posterior clinoids in the region of the foramen magnum. (Ref. 5, p. 214)

617. D. The anterior profile projection (Arcelin method) is a reverse Stenvers. (Ref. 3, p. 422)

618. B. The Stenvers projection utilizes the midsagittal plane and the infraorbitomeatal lines. (Ref. 3, p. 420)

619. C. The parietoacanthial projection of the paranasal sinuses places the orbitomeatal at a 37° angle with the plane of the film. (Ref. 5, p. 263)

620. D. The Stenvers position also demonstrates the tympanic cavity and the bony labyrinth. (Ref. 3, p. 421)

621. A. The subarachnoid space is the membrane located between the arachnoid membrane and the pia mater. (Ref. 34, p. 1760)

622. B. The trauma routine for patients with severe neck injury is to expose and check a cross-table lateral prior to moving the head or neck. (Ref. 5, p. 318)

623. B. Paranasal sinuses are located in the maxillary, frontal, ethmoid, and sphenoid bones. (Ref. 5, p. 247)

624. B. Amphiarthrodial, or slightly movable, joints are found at the intervertebral tibiofibular, sacroiliac, and symphysis pubis joints. (Ref. 5, p. 14)

625. A. The temporomandibular joint is diarthrodial, or freely movable. (Ref. 5, p. 14)

626. D. In cardiac circulation, blood returns to the heart via the four pulmonary veins that empty into the left atrium. (Ref. 37, p. 576)

627. A. At about the level of the fourth lumbar vertebra, the abdominal aorta divides into right and left common iliac arteries. (Ref. 37, p. 624)

628. C. Blood enters the liver from two sources: the hepatic artery delivers oxygenated blood from the systemic circulation; the hepatic portal vein delivers deoxygenated blood from the digestive organs. (Ref. 37, p. 621)

629. C. The abdominal aorta branches off into the right and left common iliacs at the level of L4-5 interspace. (Ref. 37, p. 624)

630. D. The two brachiocephalic veins join at a site that is immediately inferior to the first rib cartilage and close to the right sternal margin, to form the superior vena cava. (Ref. 37, p. 576)

631. A. The anterior cerebral is clearly demonstrated in the AP carotid arteriogram. (Ref. 30, p. 104)

632. D. The innominate, or brachiocephalic, trunk provides circulation to the right side of the upper extremity and head. (Ref. 34, p. 919)

633. C.   The trachea branches into the right and left bronchi at the level of D4-5. (Ref. 5, p. 39)

634. B.   The blood flows from the right cardiac ventricle through to the lungs to be oxygenated, and then back to the left cardiac atrium.

635. A.   The common hepatic duct joins the cystic duct from the gall-bladder. The two tubes become the common bile duct. (Ref. 5, p. 427)

636. B.   The sigmoid colon begins at the left iliac crest, projects inward to the midline, and terminates at the rectum at about the level of the third sacral vertebrae. (Ref. 5, p. 396)

637. D.   A good contrast abdomen film should demonstrate these areas. (Ref. 5, p. 62)

638. C.   Any study in which a perforation could exist requires careful consideration. $BaSO_4$ should not be administered. (Ref. 5, p. 402)

639. C.   Posterior obliques of 30° to 35° place the kidneys parallel with the TT. (Ref. 5, p. 445)

640. D.   Ureteric compression should not be used also in cases of recent abdominal surgery, pain, or trauma. (Ref. 5, p. 455)

641. A.   Uremia is a condition of the blood in which toxic levels of urea result in severe malfunction of the kidneys. (Ref. 17, p. 1214)

642. A.   Retrograde urography is a nonfunctional urological study. (Ref. 5, p. 457)

643. D.   Ureteric compression is utilized to enhance filling of the pelvicalyceal system and to retain the contrast media within the kidneys. (Ref. 5, p. 455)

644. B.   T-tube cholangiography is performed 6 to 8 days after a chole-cystectomy. The common bile duct may be clearly seen via direct injection or concentration of a contrast media administered via a vein. (Ref. 5, p. 433)

645. C. The female body contains two uterine (fallopian) tubes, also called oviducts, that extend laterally from the uterus and transport the ova from the ovaries to the uterus. (Ref. 37, p. 894)

646. B. The medulla contains three vital reflex centers: the cardiac center regulates heartbeat; the medullary rhythmicity area adjusts the rhythm of breathing; and the vasoconstrictor center regulates the diameter of blood vessels. (Ref. 37, p. 392)

647. D. A cystogram involves the injection of an aqueous iodine contrast medium into the bladder through a urinary catheter. (Ref. 13, p. 198)

648. B. Neo-Cholex is a cholecystagog or gallbladder stimulant. (Ref. 13, p. 207)

649. C. Hysterosalpingography and pelvic pneumography are exams to determine oviduct patency on childless women. (Ref. 5, p. 566)

650. B. Hysterosalpingography can also be performed to delineate such lesions as polyps, submucous tumor masses, and fistulous tracts. (Ref. 3, p. 183)

651. B. Cholecystocholangiography will demonstrate the gallbladder and bile duct system. (Ref. 3, p. 47)

652. B. The scout film has considerable technical value; but, if stones are visualized, the examination is usually terminated. (Ref. 13, p. 207)

653. A. The pancreatic enzymes flow into the duodenum to effect their part of the hydrolytic actions of digestion. (Ref. 37, p. 754)

654. A. The asthenic build is extremely slender and the gallbladder and stomach are both low vertical and near midline of the spine. (Ref. 3, p. 40)

655. B. An IVC study opacifies the biliary duct system. (Ref. 3, p. 54)

656. C. The right lateral decubitus position allows stones that are lighter than bile to stratify. (Ref. 3, p. 65)

657. B. Bile is either carried to the gallbladder via the cystic duct for temporary storage or poured directly into the duodenum by way of the common bile duct. (Ref. 5, p. 427)

658. B. Left and right posterior obliques demonstrate the colic flexures. (Ref. 3, p. 127)

659. B. The gallbladder drainage position (RPO) allows the contrast media to opacify the bile ducts. (Ref. 3, p. 54)

660. A. The AP Trendelenburg and AP ureteric compression positions enhance pelvicalyceal filling. (Ref. 5, p. 464)

661. D. The urethra can be well demonstrated by the voiding cystourethrogram. (Ref. 5, p. 458)

662. A. In the hypersthenic body build, the gallbladder is higher and more to the right, and the stomach is also very high and assumes a transverse position. (Ref. 5, p. 362)

663. C. Optimal visualization of the bile ducts for an IVC occurs 40 to 80 minutes after the start of the infusion. (Ref. 5, p. 432)

664. D. Cholecystopaques are usually ingested by way of 4 to 6 tablets or capsules the evening preceding the examination. (Ref. 5, p. 429)

665. B. Esophageal varices are dilated esophageal veins. They are a typical complication of portal hypertension, resulting from cirrhosis of the liver. (Ref. 7, p. 207)

666. C. In the LPO position for the upper GI, the stomach will be located higher, which requires the centering to move one vertebral body cephalad. (Ref. 5, p. 386)

667. C. The fundus, in addition to being the most superior portion of the stomach, is located posterior to the body. The pyloric portion is directed toward the posterior. (Ref. 5, p. 358)

668. D. The ileum makes up approximately three-fifths of the small bowel. (Ref. 5, p. 393)

669. B. A 35° to 45° LPO position (left AP oblique) is taken primarily to demonstrate the right colic (hepatic) flexure and the sigmoid colon. (Ref. 3, p. 126)

670. A. The right anterior oblique position in the upper GI clearly demonstrates the stomach and duodenum with barium in the distal stomach and duodenal bulb. (Ref. 5, p. 383)

671. D. The lesser curve of the stomach is the single most common site for gastric ulcers. (Ref. 7, p. 232)

672. B. The cardiac orifice is located between the esophagus and stomach, and is guarded by a circular sphincter muscle. (Ref. 5, p. 63)

673. B. A hiatal hernia can be demonstrated by placing the patient in the Trendelenburg position during an upper GI. (Ref. 3, p. 100)

674. A. A mass behind the stomach can best be demonstrated by the lateral position during the upper GI. (Ref. 5, p. 385)

675. D. In the supine position, barium will travel to the fundus, while air will locate toward the distal end of the stomach. (Ref. 5, p. 359)

676. D. The left lateral decubitus position shows accumulations of gas or free intraabdominal air under the right hemidiaphragm. (Ref. 5, p. 76)

677. B. The RAO of the barium-filled stomach will demonstrate barium in the distal stomach and duodenum. (Ref. 5, p. 383)

678. D. The ureters enter into the posterolateral portion of each side of the urinary bladder. (Ref. 5, p. 446)

679. B. The union of the major calyces is called the renal pelvis. (Ref. 37, p. 828)

680. B. A dosage of 30 to 100 mL of contrast media is administered to adults for urography. (Ref. 3, p. 152)

681. B. The descending limb of Henle dips into the medulla. It consists of squamous epithelium. There are also the u-shaped loop of Henle and an ascending limb of Henle within the medulla. (Ref. 37, p. 829)

682. C. A 30° RPO for the male patient having a voiding cystourethrogram will demonstrate the urinary bladder and urethra. (Ref. 5, p. 467)

683. A. The splenic, renal, hepatic, and celiac axies are demonstrated by abdominal aortography. (Ref. 3, p. 133)

684. B. ERCP is useful in diagnosis of biliary duct and pancreatic pathologic conditions. (Ref. 3, p. 75)

685. C. Retrograde pyelography is a follow-up study to excretory urography. (Ref. 5, p. 465)

686. B. Cholografin is administered IV for intravenous cholangiography. (Ref. 5, p. 432)

687. D. About 80% of all choleliths are of mixed combinations of cholesterol, bile pigment (bilirubin), and calcium salts. Only about 10% contain enough calcium to be radiopaque. (Ref. 24, p. 160)

688. C. Angiography requires a vessel puncture and is a strict aseptic procedure. (Ref. 5, p. 488)

689. B. In order to demonstrate very small structures in breast tissue, a fractional focal spot is required. (Ref. 3, p. 64)

690. C. Glucagon, a product of alpha cells, accelerates the conversion of glycogen into glucose in the liver. (Ref. 37, p. 499)

691. D. Hirschsprung's disease is a loss of peristalsis and paralytic obstruction, particularly of the rectum and rectosigmoid colon. (Ref. 7, p. 312)

692. D. Lower extremity venograms demonstrate the circulatory patterns of the legs. (Ref. 3, p. 145)

693. B. The mediolateral of a well-compressed breast shows glandular and fatty tissue, with the nipple in profile. (Ref. 5, p. 350)

694. D. The purpose of arthrography is to demonstrate all junctions between bones or between cartilage and bones. (Ref. 30, p. 194)

695. D. In translumbar aortography, a 6- to 8-in translumbar needle is passed percutaneously into the abdominal aorta. (Ref. 3, p. 131)

696. D. A delayed film of 24 hours is the phase of the study called lymphadenography. (Ref. 30, p. 174)

697. B. In order to maintain contrast xeromammography, films are taken in the high 40- to 50-kVp level. (Ref. 3, p. 62)

698. C. A lumbar puncture is usually performed between the third and the fourth lumbar vertebra for opaque myelography. (Ref. 3, p. 102)

699. B. When performing abdominal aortography, the central ray is usually directed to the level of L-2, and the exposures are made at the end of suspended respiration. (Ref. 3, p. 134)

700. B. The puncture is made at L2-3 or L3-4 interspace, or at the cisterna cerebello medullaris. The cord ends at L-2. (Ref. 3, p. 102)

5 Patient Care and Management

The major subject areas covered in patient care and management include the following.

1. Medico-legal implications, scheduling, informed consent, patient rights, liability, patient identification, interpretation of request form, clinical observations and information, and processing of examination requisition.

2. Nursing procedures involving patient safety and comfort, including body mechanics, methods of communication, assessment of condition, safety in dealing with attached equipment, ethical principles, and documentation of events.

3. Sterile techniques procedures involving hand washing, contamination, gowning, gloving and masking, syringes, sterile supplies, and disposal procedures.

4. Injectable and noninjectable contrast media agents; contraindications; adverse reactions; radiologic emergencies; first aid; CPR; communicable diseases; patient assessment; instructions for contrast examinations; administration of contrast agents; and monitoring of medical equipment, including catheters, oxygen, and common medical instrumentation.

5. Vital signs application, including blood pressure monitoring, pulse, respiration, and usage of equipment.

6. Dealing with isolation patients, including disinfectant procedures, approach, and equipment usage.

DIRECTIONS (Questions 701–800): Each of the questions or incomplete statements below is followed by four suggested answers or completions. Select the **one** that is best in each case.

701. If an invasive procedure is being prepared and the radiographer finds that the consent form has not been signed, he/she should
    A. call the floor after the procedure
    B. inform the radiologist prior to injection
    C. continue with the preparation
    D. administer antiallergenic medications

702. If the radiographer left a sick patient unattended and he/she fell off the x-ray table and sustained a serious injury, the radiographer could be sued for
    A. battery
    B. negligence
    C. reasonable care
    D. felony

703. Which of the following procedures would require an operative consent form?
    1. Arteriogram
    2. Myelogram
    3. Pneumoencephalogram
    A. 1 only
    B. 2 only
    C. 1 and 3 only
    D. 1, 2, and 3

704. A radiographer would be negligent if he/she
    A. committed an illegal act against society
    B. failed to give reasonable care
    C. unlawfully handled a person without his consent
    D. threatened to injure another person

705. The patient may be able to respond to all stimuli, but is confused about reality with respect to persons, time, place, or events. This level of consciousness is called
 A. unconscious
 B. semiconscious
 C. disoriented
 D. conscious

706. A patient's consent to or refusal of services may be
  1. written
  2. oral
  3. implied
 A. 1 only
 B. 1 and 2 only
 C. 2 and 3 only
 D. 1, 2, and 3

707. If a patient asks the radiographer about the results of his examination, he/she should be
 A. told to ask the radiologist
 B. informed of the findings
 C. assured that the referring physician will be informed
 D. referred to the chief technologist

708. When a trauma patient experiences a rapid heartbeat with low blood pressure and lacks normal color, he/she is experiencing
 A. signs of shock
 B. ataxia
 C. eclampsia
 D. lethargy

709. A *normal* response to the injection of an iodine contrast media is a
  1. warm flushed feeling
  2. metallic taste
  3. pain at the injection site
 A. 1 and 2 only
 B. 1 and 3 only
 C. 2 and 3 only
 D. 1, 2, and 3

710. If a patient feels faint, the radiographer should
   A. administer smelling salts
   B. lie the patient down and elevate his/her legs
   C. return the patient to a wheelchair
   D. sit the patient up and administer oxygen

711. If a patient experiences an epileptic seizure, the primary concern of the radiographer is to
   1. protect the patient from injury
   2. establish an airway
   3. restrain the patient
   A. 1 only
   B. 1 and 2 only
   C. 2 and 3 only
   D. 1, 2, and 3

712. Which of the following drugs is a cardiotonic?
   A. Erythromycin
   B. Meprobamate
   C. Benadryl
   D. Digitalis

713. Heparin is used in radiography studies to
   A. eliminate pain
   B. increase urine output
   C. increase coagulation
   D. decrease coagulation

714. Which of the following **BEST** describes the term *extravasation?*
   A. Imbalance in fluid levels
   B. Fluid escaping from vessels
   C. Aversion to blood
   D. Excessive urinary output

715. In preparation for a contrast media study of the gastrointestinal tract, the patient should have
A. 10 to 20 cc of Pontocaine
B. 2 oz castor oil prior to the exam
C. iodine skin test
D. barium allergy test

716. The term *hematemesis* refers to
A. blood effusion into a cavity
B. a blood cyst
C. coagulation of the blood
D. vomiting of blood

717. If a patient experiences urticaria following the injection of a contrast agent, the radiologist will then administer a
A. adrenergic
B. antipyretic
C. antihistamine
D. prochlorperazine

718. When moving a patient from the supine to the prone position, the radiographer should **ALWAYS** turn the patient
A. away from himself
B. the longest distance
C. toward himself
D. toward the weak side

719. Which type of shock occurs from a severe allergic reaction to an injected contrast media?
A. Septic
B. Anaphylactic
C. Cardiogenic
D. Hypovolemic

720. Which of the following is an example of a communicable disease?
A. Gastroenteritis
B. Pneumonia
C. Dysphagia
D. Nephritis

721. When a drug requires a quick response, it should be administered
   A. intracavitary
   B. intramuscularly
   C. orally
   D. intravenously

722. If a contrast media extravasates from the injection site, the technologist should
   A. cover the site with a bandage and elevate the patient's feet
   B. turn the patient on his/her side
   C. apply a warm towel over the injection site
   D. prepare a syringe containing an antihistamine

723. Patients with blood pressure diastolic readings of 110 or higher are classified as
   A. neurogenic
   B. hypertensive
   C. cardiogenic
   D. antitussive

724. If an IV becomes infiltrated, the radiographer should immediately
   A. increase the flow
   B. stop the flow of solution
   C. decrease the height of the bottle
   D. raise the height to 20 in

725. Which of the following examinations does **NOT** require the patient to be NPO?
   A. Small bowel series
   B. Esophagram
   C. Lower GI series
   D. Gallbladder series

726. Which of the following conditions would relate to an intravenous urography examination?
1. Wilms' tumor
2. Pyelonephritis
3. Hematuria
 A. 1 only
 B. 1 and 2 only
 C. 2 and 3 only
 D. 1, 2, and 3

727. If a radiograph is ordered "stat," it means
 A. whenever necessary
 B. immediately
 C. after meals
 D. at bedtime

728. If a patient experiences a convulsion seizure, the radiographer should
 A. apply cold compresses to the forehead
 B. elevate the feet
 C. administer medication
 D. prevent the patient from injury

729. Patients undergoing an upper GI series should be NPO for approximately
 A. 2 to 3 hours
 B. five hours
 C. 8 to 10 hours
 D. 24 hours

730. Which of the following medications will dilate blood vessels?
 A. Digitalis
 B. Nitroglycerine
 C. Aminophyllin
 D. Demerol

731. Which of the following drugs is an antibacterial?
   A. Emetic
   B. Antibiotic
   C. Diuretic
   D. Analgesic

732. Which of the following abbreviations is stated **INCORRECTLY?**
   A. BID: twice a day
   B. TID: three times a day
   C. QID: four times a day
   D. Q2H: every four hours

733. In order to properly transfer a patient from a wheelchair to the x-ray table, the technologist should
   1. explain the task clearly
   2. assist the patient
   3. allow the patient to move unassisted
   A. 1 only
   B. 1 and 2 only
   C. 2 and 3 only
   D. 1, 2, and 3

734. A condition free of contamination or germs is called
   A. anoxic
   B. aseptic
   C. astringent
   D. aerobic

735. Which of the following statements regarding sterile technique is **INCORRECT?**
   A. Avoid reaching over a sterile field
   B. A sterile article is handled with a sterile instrument or sterile gloves
   C. Only the outside of a wrapper is touched when opening a sterile package or container
   D. Pour sterile solutions with contact between the bottle and sides of the container to avoid spillage

736. The **MOST** common reason for an IV to stop dripping is
  A. infusion
  B. infiltration
  C. clogged tubing
  D. blockage

737. Which of the following is considered a mild reaction to the injection of an iodinated contrast media?
  A. Vasovagal response
  B. Tachycardia
  C. Hypotension
  D. Laryngeal edema

738. The word that **BEST** describes the escape of fluid into a part of tissue is
  A. infiltration
  B. effusion
  C. infusion
  D. distention

739. Air bubbles can usually be differentiated from radiolucent stones in the biliary tract because
  A. air bubbles are smaller than stones
  B. stones have a smooth, spherical shape
  C. air bubbles will move with each injection of contrast media
  D. most stones are radiopaque

740. Which of the following needles would **MOST** probably be used for injecting a child for an IVP?
  A. 14 gauge
  B. 16 gauge
  C. 18 gauge
  D. 25 gauge

741. Which exam does **NOT** require strict aseptic technique?
  A. Myelography
  B. Pacemaker
  C. Upper GI series
  D. Arteriography

742. The **MOST** common injection site for an **IV** contrast media examination is the
  A. saphenous vein
  B. antecubital vein
  C. radial vein
  D. popliteal vein

743. A common procedure performed on nongravid patients is a
  A. laparotomy
  B. hysterosalpingogram
  C. fetography
  D. cystourethrogram

744. If an **IV** infiltrates, the technologist should
  A. readjust the needle
  B. increase the flow rate
  C. slow it down and have it checked
  D. apply mild compression

745. In order to properly inflate a Bardex retention tip, the amount of air required is
  A. 30 cc
  B. 50 cc
  C. 90 cc
  D. 120 cc

746. Viscosity refers to a contrast media's
  1. iodine content
  2. thickness
  3. opacity
  A. 1 only
  B. 2 only
  C. 1 and 3 only
  D. 1, 2, and 3

747. An adult patient with abnormal rapidity of heart action, usually over 100 beats per minute at rest, is experiencing
    A. hypotension
    B. tachycardia
    C. hyperventilation
    D. apnea

748. Normal adult body temperature, measured orally, is
    A. 96.0 °F
    B. 98.6 °F
    C. 99.2 °F
    D. 99.8 °F

749. Syncope may be caused by
    1. vagal stimulation
    2. diaphoresis
    3. emotional stress
    A. 1 only
    B. 1 and 2 only
    C. 2 and 3 only
    D. 1, 2, and 3

750. The normal number of pulse beats per minute in the average adult is
    A. 60 to 80
    B. 80 to 100
    C. 100 to 120
    D. 120 to 150

751. Which of the following vital signs is abnormal for the adult patient?
    A. Blood pressure 100/60
    B. Temperature (oral) 98 °F to 99 °F
    C. Pulse 110 beats/min
    D. Respirations 12 to 16/min

752. The easiest way to open the airway is to
    A. sit the patient up
    B. tilt the patient's head back
    C. strike the patient on the back
    D. turn the head to one side

753. Cardiac compressions for an adult during CPR should be administered at a rate of
    A. 30 to 45/min
    B. 60/min
    C. 80 to 120/min
    D. 140 to 160/min

754. During CPR, which of the following drugs is usually administered?
    A. Epinephrine
    B. Heparin
    C. Atropine
    D. Neo-Cholex

755. The artery **MOST** commonly used to check a person's pulse is the
    A. pedal
    B. radial
    C. brachial
    D. popliteal

756. Orthopnea refers to
    A. discomfort in breathing
    B. air within the pericardium
    C. rapid breathing
    D. abnormal gas in the pleura

757. Which of the following would **NOT** be a sign of shock?
    A. Vertigo
    B. Pallor
    C. Anxiety
    D. Uremia

758. Systolic pressure is considered elevated when it continually exceeds
   A. 80
   B. 90
   C. 140
   D. 160

759. The contraction phase of the heart is known as
   A. cardiodilation
   B. systole
   C. pulse
   D. diastole

760. A reading of 65 to 80 mm of mercury is normal for
   A. systolic pressure
   B. diastolic pressure
   C. portal pressure
   D. femoral pressure

761. When performing a cross-table lateral position of the cervical spine, the central ray is directed to
   A. C-2
   B. C-3
   C. C-4
   D. C-6

762. An escaping of blood that causes discoloration of the surrounding tissues is referred to as
   A. edema
   B. exostosis
   C. ecchymosis
   D. effusion

763. When a patient reacts to an intravenous injection, the radiographer should immediately
   A. attach oxygen
   B. elevate the head
   C. send for the doctor
   D. inject Benadryl

764. A patient who has lost a considerable amount of blood due to an open wound is susceptible to shock termed
  A. anaphylactic
  B. hypovolemic
  C. septic
  D. cardiogenic

765. Enteric isolation requires that the radiographer use
  A. no special precautions
  B. gloves and a gown
  C. a surgical gown and boots
  D. a mask and gown

766. If a patient begins to experience vertigo and syncope, the technologist should
  A. begin CPR
  B. turn the patient's head to the side
  C. lie the patient down
  D. administer medication

767. Stroke patients may also suffer from
  A. dysoxia
  B. dysphonia
  C. dysplasia
  D. dysphagia

768. Which of the following occur during cardiac arrest?
    1. Heart beat and pulse are absent
    2. Circulation stops
    3. Pupils of the eyes gradually dilate
  A. 1 only
  B. 2 only
  C. 1 and 3 only
  D. 1, 2, and 3

769. When a patient's heart has stopped beating and the blood no longer circulates through the body, he/she is experiencing cardiac
   A. tamponade
   B. arrest
   C. apnea
   D. arrhythmia

770. The condition that exists when fluids are collected in tissue due to an improperly placed needle in a vein is called a(an)
   A. infusion
   B. infiltrate
   C. intracellular
   D. irrigation

771. The adult adapts **BEST** to IV fluids administered at a drops per minute steady rate of
   A. 10 to 20
   B. 20 to 60
   C. 60 to 100
   D. 100 to 150

772. During shock, the patient should be
   A. administered external heat
   B. given medication by mouth
   C. given IV fluids to restore blood volume
   D. placed in the Trendelenburg position

773. Which of the following drugs can be administered to a patient experiencing anaphylactic shock?
   1. Subcutaneous epinephrine
   2. Corticosteroids
   3. IV diphenhydramine
   A. 1 only
   B. 1 and 2 only
   C. 2 and 3 only
   D. 1, 2, and 3

774. Approximately how far must the urinary catheter be inserted into the female patient before urine begins to flow?
   A. 5 to 6 cm
   B. 7 to 8 cm
   C. 8 to 10 cm
   D. 11 to 12 cm

775. During CPR, the compression/ventilation (C/V) ratio for two rescuers on older children and adults is
   A. 100 c/20 v/min
   B. 80 c/15 v/min
   C. 60 c/12 v/min
   D. 40 c/10 v/min

776. How far should the sternum be depressed for chest compressions performed on an adult during CPR?
   A. 0.5 to 1 in
   B. 1.5 to 2 in
   C. 2.5 to 3 in
   D. 3.5 to 4 in

777. A patient going into shock would have the early signs of
   1. fall in blood pressure
   2. pale, clammy skin
   3. rapid, thready pulse
   A. 1 only
   B. 1 and 2 only
   C. 2 and 3 only
   D. 1, 2, and 3

778. Within 20 to 40 seconds after cardiac arrest, a person is considered
   A. brain dead
   B. clinically dead
   C. cardiac dead
   D. respiratory dead

779. During cardiac arrest, if respiratory arrest occurs first and the heart continues to beat, the
  1. femoral pulse should be palpated
  2. skin color will be cyanotic
  3. patient can be administered oxygen

  A. 1 only
  B. 2 only
  C. 1 and 3 only
  D. 1, 2, and 3

780. The long plastic or rubber tube used to drain stomach fluids is called a
  A. gomcothermotic tube
  B. Levin tube
  C. cantor tube
  D. Miller-Abbott tube

781. The GI tube with an inflatable rubber bag used to drain or decompress the small intestine is called a
  A. Miller-Abbott tube
  B. Rehfuss tube
  C. Ewald tube
  D. Jutte tube

782. A common preoperative drug for bronchography is
  A. Chlor-Trimeton
  B. Lasix
  C. heparin
  D. atropine

783. Which of the following solutions is nonopaque?
  A. Bilopaque
  B. Saline
  C. Hypaque
  D. Ethiodol

784. Which of the following examinations could cause complications for a patient allergic to seafood?
A. Pyelography and angiography
B. Hysterosalpingography
C. Pneumoencephalography
D. Thermography

785. If the chance exists that a patient will have surgery immediately following a barium enema, the contrast media induced will be
A. barium sulphate single contrast
B. water-soluble single contrast
C. water-soluble and air double contrast
D. barium sulphate and air double contrast

786. Cathartics are used to
A. induce vomiting
B. cleanse the colon
C. prevent nausea
D. dilate vessels

787. The contrast media **MOST** commonly used in myelography is
A. oil based
B. a barium sulphate suspension
C. one that prevents nausea
D. water-soluble iodinated

788. Which of the following reactions to contrast media would **NOT** be considered mild?
A. Urticaria
B. Nausea
C. Dyspnea
D. Sneezing

789. Which of the following conditions requires an **INCREASE** in technical factors?
A. Osteoma
B. Blastomycosis
C. Fibrosarcoma
D. Osteoporosis

790. Which disease(s) require(s) a **DECREASE** in exposure factors?
    1. Osteoporosis
    2. Pleural effusion
    3. Emphysema
  A. 1 and 2 only
  B. 1 and 3 only
  C. 2 and 3 only
  D. 1, 2, and 3

791. Which of the following chest pathological conditions would require a **DECREASE** in technique from a "normal" chest?
  A. Atelectasis
  B. Pneumothorax
  C. Pleural effusion
  D. Pneumonia

792. Which of the following skeletal pathological conditions **INCREASES** bone opacity and requires an increase in technical factors?
  A. Fibrosarcoma
  B. Osteochondroma
  C. Hemangioma
  D. Neuroblastoma

793. During cardiac arrest, the patient is intravenously administered a drug to combat acidosis called
  A. Phenergan
  B. sodium bicarbonate
  C. hydrocortisone
  D. sodium chloride

794. A disease that a patient contracts within the hospital is termed
  A. pathogenic
  B. contact
  C. nosocomial
  D. enteric

795. Isolation units required for severe burn patients are termed
  A. contact
  B. strict
  C. protective
  D. enteric

796. When a patient is scheduled for a GI series, he/she should be NPO prior to the exam for at **LEAST**
  A. 5 to 6 hours
  B. 8 to 12 hours
  C. 14 to 16 hours
  D. 24 hours

797. What is the order followed for contrast exams performed in the morning?
  1. Barium enema
  2. Upper GI
  3. IVP
  A. 1, 2, and 3
  B. 3, 1, and 2
  C. 2, 3, and 1
  D. 3, 2, and 1

798. If the patient is placed on the x-ray table for an IVP examination, where should the urinary drainage bag be positioned?
  A. On the table
  B. Secured on an IV pole
  C. In contact with the bladder
  D. Below the level of the bladder

799. Which of the following drugs is administered as a vasodilator?
  A. Nitroglycerine
  B. Cholorothiazide
  C. Heparin
  D. Reserpine

800. Which of the following types of medical equipment is raised above the level of the patient and table top?
   1. Urinary catheters and bag
   2. Intravenous solutions
   3. Abdominal drainage tube
A. 1 only
B. 2 only
C. 1 and 3 only
D. 1, 2, and 3

Explanatory Answers

701. B. The radiographer especially must not proceed with an invasive procedure without written consent. (Ref. 13, p. 15)

702. B. Negligence is the failing to perform some act that a reasonably prudent person would carry out in a similar circumstance. (Ref. 27, p. 24)

703. D. All surgical procedures and biopsies require that an operative consent be signed preoperatively. (Ref. 27, p. 104)

704. B. Negligence occurs when the radiographer takes the wrong action and/or fails to act reasonably. (Ref. 27, p. 24)

705. C. During the disoriented stage, speech often is irrelevant and behavior may be inappropriate. (Ref. 27, p. 604)

706. D. A patient's consent may be written, oral, or implied. Written consent is preferred because it is easier to prove. (Ref. 27, p. 100)

707. C. The patient has a right to be informed accurately about his treatment; however, the radiographer may not divulge the results of a diagnostic test. (Ref. 36, p. 4)

708. A. General signs and symptoms of shock include decreased temperature; a weak, thready pulse; a rapid heartbeat; rapid shallow respirations; hypotension; skin pallor; cyanosis; and increased thirst. (Ref. 36, p. 76)

709. D. All three responses are symptoms of mild reactions to iodinated contrast agents. (Ref. 36, p. 201)

710. B. If a patient experiences syncope, or fainting, he/she should be placed in a dorsal recumbant position with the feet elevated. (Ref. 13, p. 158)

711. A. The radiographer should protect the patient from injury and carefully note the sequence of seizure activity without administering severe restraint. (Ref. 17, p. 434)

712. D. Digitalis is a cardiotonic prescribed in the treatment of congestive heart failure and certain cardiac arrhythmias. (Ref. 17, p. 371)

713. D. Heparin sodium is an anticoagulant prescribed in the treatment of a variety of thromboembolic disorders. (Ref. 17, p. 560)

714. B. Extravasation is a passage or escape into the tissues, usually of blood, serum, or lymph. (Ref. 17, p. 456)

715. B. Castor oil given prior to the upper GI exam will assist in demonstrating the organ empty. (Ref. 5, p. 368)

716. D. Hematemesis is the vomiting of bright, red blood, indicating rapid upper GI bleeding. (Ref. 17, p. 553)

717. C. An intermediate reaction such as urticaria (hives) is treated by the administration of an antihistamine such as Benedryl. (Ref. 13, p. 160)

718. C. In utilizing the log roll, the patient is turned toward the radiographer. (Ref. 36, p. 46)

719. B. Anaphylactic shock is due to extreme sensitivity to a drug, person, or foreign substance. (Ref. 13, p. 161)

720. B. Pneumonia is an acute inflammation of the lungs, usually caused by inhaled pneumococci. (Ref. 17, p. 933)

721. D. Administration of drugs IV is the fastest route during emergencies. (Ref. 36, p. 187)

722. C. Mild reactions can occur at the injection site by extravasation. A warm towel placed over the injection site may speed absorption of the contrast medium. (Ref. 5, p. 452)

723. B. Patients with blood pressure exceeding 140/90 mm HG are classified as hypertensive. (Ref. 13, p. 87)

724. B. If the IV site is cool, swollen, and boggy, the IV may have infiltrated, and the radiologist should be notified. (Ref. 13, p. 135)

725. B. Since the esophagus is empty most of the time, there is no need for patient preparation unless an upper GI series is to follow. (Ref. 5, p. 386)

726. D. All three conditions relate to the urinary tract. (Ref. 13, p. 198)

727. B. If a x-ray exam is requested "stat" it means that it should be performed immediately. (Ref. 36, p. 192)

728. D. The correct action for a patient seizure is to place the patient supine and keep him secure. (Ref. 36, p. 86)

729. C. The patient should not eat anything for 8 to 10 hours prior to the upper GI. (Ref. 13, p. 171)

730. B. Nitroglycerine is a coronary vasodilator. (Ref. 17, p. 816)

731. B. Antibiotics have the ability to destroy or interfere with the development of a living organism. (Ref. 17, p. 74)

732. D. Q2H means every two hours—*not* every four hours. (Ref. 13, p. 253)

733. B. Patients must be kept positioned so that their bodies are in good alignment with the technologist and the wheelchair. They should never move unassisted. (Ref. 36, p. 46)

734. B. The aseptic is a sterile germ-free condition. (Ref. 27, p. 598)

735. D. Pour sterile solutions so there is no contact between the bottle and the sides of the container. (Ref. 18, p. 118)

736. B. The IV will stop dripping when the needle is not properly placed in the vein. (Ref. 27, p. 661)

737. A. A vasovagal response of fear, with signs of weakness, dizziness, and sweating, is a mild reaction. (Ref. 5, p. 452)

738. B. Effusion is the escape of fluid from blood vessels because of rupture or seepage, usually into a body cavity. (Ref. 17, p. 406)

739. C. Residual stones will not move as freely as air bubbles when performing a postoperative cholangiography. (Ref. 3, p. 72)

740. D. The needle with the smallest lumen (25 gauge) would be used for a small injection into a small vessel. (Ref. 38, p. 102)

741. C. Procedures requiring injection call for sterile technique. When contrast media is ingested, strict sterile technique is not required. (Ref. 13, p. 168)

742. B. The antecubital vein, located at the bend of the anterior elbow, is an ideal IV injection site. (Ref. 13, p. 128)

743. B. Hysterosalpingography delineates the uterine cavity and lumen of the tubal passages. (Ref. 3, p. 183)

744. C. Infiltration occurs when a fluid passes into the tissue such as via a misplaced IV needle. (Ref. 13, p. 134)

745. C. A reusable squeeze inflator is recommended to limit the air capacity to approximately 90 cc. (Ref. 3, p. 111)

746. B. Viscosity relates to the thickness of the contrast medium. (Ref. 30, p. 198)

747. B. Tachycardia in adults is over 100 beats per minute at rest; for children it is over 200 beats per minute. (Ref. 27, p. 182)

748. B. Oral temperatures ranging from 96.5 °F to 99 °F are consistent with good health. 98.6 °F is normal adult body temperature measured orally. (Ref. 27, p. 404)

749. D. Syncope, or fainting, is a sensation of light-headedness that can be treated by lying down or by sitting with the head between the knees. (Ref. 17, p. 1142)

750. A. Rates of 60 to 80 pulse beats per minute for an adult and 120 pulse beats per minute for a newborn are average. (Ref. 17, p. 988)

751. C. A rapid pulse called tachycardia exists when over 100 beats per minute are recorded. (Ref. 13, p. 76)

752. B. To open the airway, tilt the patient's head back by placing one hand under the neck and lifting it. (Ref. 27, p. 554)

753. B. A rate of 60 cardiac compressions and 12 assisted respirations per minute are required for an adult patient during CPR. (Ref. 17, p. 205)

754. A. Epinephrine is administered during CPR, along with sodium bicarbonate and calcium chloride. (Ref. 36, p. 208)

755. B. A common pulse point is the radial artery in the wrist, at the base of the thumb. (Ref. 27, p. 416)

756. A. Orthopnea is an abnormal condition in which a person must sit or stand in order to breathe deeply or comfortably. (Ref. 17, p. 849)

757. D. Uremia relates to the presence of excessive amounts of urea in the blood and is unrelated to shock. (Ref. 17, p. 1214)

758. C. The average blood pressure in a healthy young adult is considered to be 120/80 mm of mercury. Systolic pressure above 140 is outside the normal range. (Ref. 27, p. 425)

759. B. The systolic is the first sound heard as blood enters the collapsed vein. (Ref. 27, p. 404)

760. B. A reading of 65 to 80 mm of mercury is normal diastolic pressure for a young, healthy adult. (Ref. 27, p. 425)

761. C. A good cross-table lateral of the cervical spine should demonstrate all seven cervical vertebrae. (Ref. 5, p. 318)

762. C. Ecchymosis is a discoloration of an area of the skin by extravasation of blood. (Ref. 17, p. 401)

763. C. Should a patient have an allergic reaction, the technologist should immediately notify the radiologist. (Ref. 36, p. 78)

764. B. Hypovolemic shock is caused by an abnormally low volume of circulating fluid (plasma) in the body. (Ref. 13, p. 154)

765. B. For enteric isolation cases, protective gowns are worn if soiling is possible, as are gloves if infected material may be touched. (Ref. 36, p. 29)

766. C. If a patient begins to have an allergic reaction, the technologist should stop the radiographic exam and place the patient in a supine position. (Ref. 36, p. 85)

767. B. Dysphonia is the inability to speak and is closely associated with stroke patients. (Ref. 34, p. 547)

768. D. When cardiac arrest occurs, the heartbeat and pulse are absent, blood pressure falls to zero, respirations cease, and the pupils begin to dilate. (Ref. 27, p. 552)

769. B. When cardiac arrest occurs, the heart stops beating from a lack of sufficient oxygen to the heart muscle. (Ref. 27, p. 552)

770. B. Infiltrates occur when the needle is not properly placed in the vein, causing a collection of fluid in the tissue. (Ref. 27, p. 61)

771. B. A steady rate of 20 to 60 regular drops per minute, or 80 to 250 mL per hour, is ideal for adult IV therapy. (Ref. 27, p. 667)

772. C. Blood volume must be restored quickly so that there can be a rapid return of oxygenated blood to the perfusion-deprived tissue. (Ref. 17, p. 1077)

773. D. Nursing care of patients experiencing anaphylactic shock requires the administration of these drugs and monitoring of blood pressure, central nervous system, and urinary output. (Ref. 17, p. 61)

774. B. A urinary catheter is inserted approximately 7.5 cm into the female meatus until the urine begins to flow. (Ref. 13, p. 202)

775. C. The compression/ventilation ratio for adults alone is 15/2, and for two rescuers 5/1, or 60 c/12 v/min. (Ref. 17, p. 204)

776. B. The sternum compression distance for an adult is 1.5 to 2 in (4 to 5 cm). (Ref. 17, p. 205)

777. D. Early signs of shock include all of the signs listed: decreased blood pressure, pale skin, and rapid pulse. (Ref. 27, p. 605)

778. B. When a victim stops breathing and loses consciousness, within 20 to 40 seconds after cardiac arrest the person is considered clinically dead. (Ref. 27, p. 552)

779. B. If respiratory arrest occurs first and the heart continues to beat, the skin color will be bluish, or cyanotic. (Ref. 36, p. 81)

780. B. The tube used to drain off fluids and decompress the stomach is called a Levin tube. (Ref. 27, p. 681)

781. A. The Miller-Abbott tube is the most common of the GI tubes used to drain or decompress the small intestine. (Ref. 27, p. 681)

782. D. Epinephrine or atropine are drugs given to minimize bronchial secretions prior to a bronchogram. (Ref. 13, p. 215)

783. B. Saline is a solution containing sodium chloride which is non-opaque. (Ref. 17, p. 1049)

784. A. The technologist should question the patient about allergies prior to an intravenous contrast injection. Iodine found in most seafoods is the base for vascular contrast mediums. (Ref. 13, p. 160)

785. B. When the possibility of surgery exists, a water-soluble single contrast agent should be utilized. (Ref. 5, p. 408)

786. B. Either irritant cathartics, such as castor oil, or saline cathartics, such as magnesium citrate and magnesium sulfate, can be used to cleanse the bowel. (Ref. 5, p. 509)

787. D. The best type of contrast medium for myelography is one that is miscible with cerebrospinal fluid. (Ref. 5, p. 560)

788. C. Dyspnea, or difficulty in breathing, is considered a severe reaction. (Ref. 5, p. 452)

789. A. Osteoma is an additive disease that requires increased penetration. (Ref. 35, p. 241)

790. A. With osteoporosis there is a loss of calcium from the bone, leaving it less dense. Emphysema is a destructive lung disease that is also easily penetrated. Both diseases require a reduction in exposure technique. (Ref. 35, p. 241)

791. B. A pneumothorax would be categorized as a destructive (easy to penetrate) condition and would, therefore, require a reduction of the normal chest radiographic technique. (Ref. 35, p. 241)

792. B. Osteochondroma would create an additive condition, which would be harder to penetrate than normal bone and cartilage. (Ref. 35, p. 241)

793. B. Sodium bicarbonate treats metabolic acidosis in cases of cardiac arrest. (Ref. 17, p. 1094)

794. C. When a patient acquires an infection while in a health care institution, it is termed a nosocomial infection. (Ref. 36. p. 18)

795. B. Strict isolation is utilized for patients who are themselves at high risk for infection, such as patients with severe burns. (Ref. 36, p. 31)

796. B. The NPO order is commonly instituted for a limited period of approximately 8 to 12 hours prior to an upper GI series. (Ref. 13, p. 171)

797. B. The order is IVP first, then gallbladder, then barium enema, then upper GI. (Ref. 13, p. 272)

798. D. The urine collection bag must be held below the level of the patient's bladder. (Ref. 13, p. 70)

799. A. Nitroglycerine is a drug that lowers blood pressure and counteracts pain due to circulatory disturbance. (Ref. 13, p. 122)

800. B. Urinary collection bags and abdominal drainage tubes must be located below the level of the patient. (Ref. 13, p. 70)

References

1. Anderson KN, Anderson LE: *Mosby's Pocket Dictionary of Medicine, Nursing, and Allied Health.* St Louis, CV Mosby Co, 1990.

2. Ballinger P: *Pocket Guide to Radiography.* St Louis, CV Mosby Co, 1989.

3. Ballinger PW: *Merrill's Atlas of Radiologic Positions and Radiologic Procedures,* ed 7. St Louis, CV Mosby Co, 1991.

4. Birmingham J: *Medical Terminology: A Self-Learning Text,* ed 2. St Louis, CV Mosby Co, 1990.

5. Bontrager K, Anthony BT: *Textbook of Radiographic Positioning and Related Anatomy,* ed 2. Denver, Multi Media, 1987.

6. Bushong SC: *Radiologic Science for Technologists: Physics, Biology, and Protection,* ed 4. St Louis, CV Mosby Co, 1988.

7. Cawson RA, McCracken A, Marcus P, Zaatari G: *Pathology: The Mechanism of Disease,* ed 2. St Louis, CV Mosby Co, 1989.

8. Cullinan J, Cullinan A: *Illustrated Guide to X-ray Techniques,* ed 2. Philadelphia, JB Lippincott, 1980.

9. Curry TS, Dowdey JE, Murry RC: *Christensen's Introduction to the Physics of Diagnostic Radiology,* ed 4. Philadelphia, Lea & Febiger, 1990.

10. De Vos D: *Basic Principles of Radiographic Exposure.* Philadelphia, Lea & Febiger, 1990.

11. Donohue DP: *An Analysis of Radiographic Quality.* Baltimore, University Park Press, 1984.

12. Drafke M: *Trauma and Mobile Radiography.* Philadelphia, FA Davis, 1990.

13. Ehrlich RA, McCloskey Givens E: *Patient Care in Radiography,* ed 3. St Louis, CV Mosby Co, 1989.

14. Eisenberg RL, Dennis C, May C: *Radiographic Positioning.* Boston, Little Brown & Co, 1989.

15. Eisenberg RL, Dennis CA: *Comprehensive Radiographic Pathology.* St Louis, CV Mosby Co, 1990.

16. *Fundamentals of Radiography,* ed 12. Rochester, NY, Medical Division, Eastman Kodak Company, 1980.

17. Glanze WD: *Mosby's Medical and Nursing Dictionary,* ed 3. St Louis, CV Mosby Co, 1990.

18. Gurley LT, Callaway WJ: *Introduction to Radiologic Technology,* ed 2. St Louis, CV Mosby Co, 1986.

19. Gylys BA, Wedding ME: *Medical Terminology: A Systems Approach.* Philadelphia, FA Davis Co, 1988.

20. Kent TH, Hart MN: *Introduction to Human Disease,* ed 2. Norwalk, CT, Appleton-Century-Croft, 1987.

21. Laudicina P: *Applied Pathology for Radiographers.* Philadelphia, WB Saunders Co, 1989.

22. Leonard PC: *Building a Medical Terminology,* ed 2. Philadelphia, WB Saunders Co, 1988.

23. Leonard PC: *Quick and Easy Medical Terminology.* Philadelphia, WB Saunders Co, 1990.

24. Mace JD, Kowalczyk N: *Radiographic Pathology for Technologists.* St Louis, CV Mosby Co, 1988.

25. Mulvihill ML: *Human Diseases—A Systemic Approach,* ed 2. Norwalk, CT, Appleton and Lange, 1987.

26. Noz ME, Maguire GQ: *Radiation Protection in the Radiologic and Health Sciences,* ed 2. Philadelphia, Lea & Febiger, 1985.

27. Rambo BJ, Wood LA: *Nursing Skills for Clinical Practice,* ed 3. Philadelphia, WB Saunders Co, 1982.

28. Rice J: *Medical Terminology with Human Anatomy,* ed 2. Norwalk, CT, Appleton and Lange, 1991.

29. Selman J: *The Fundamentals of X-ray and Radium Physics,* ed 7. Springfield, IL, Charles C Thomas, 1985.

30. Snopek A: *Fundamentals of Special Radiographic Procedures,* ed 2. Philadelphia, WB Saunders Co, 1984.

31. Statkiewicz MA, Ritenour R: *Radiation Protection for Student Radiographers.* Denver, Multi Media, 1983.

32. Swallow RA, Naylor E: *Clark's Positioning in Radiography,* ed 11. Rockville, MD, Aspen Publishers, 1986.

33. Sweeney RJ: *Radiographic Artifacts: Their Cause and Control.* Philadelphia, JB Lippincott, 1983.

34. *Taber's Cyclopedic Medical Dictionary,* ed 16. Philadelphia, FA Davis, 1989.

35. Thompson TT: *Cahoon's Formulating X-ray Techniques,* ed 9. Durham, NC, Duke University Press, 1979.

242 / Radiography

242 / Radiography

242 / Radiography

242 / Radiography

36. Torres L, Morrill C: *Basic Medical Techniques and Patient Care for Radiologic Technologists,* ed 3. Philadelphia, JB Lippincott, 1989.

37. Tortora G, Anagnostakos N: *Principles of Anatomy and Physiology,* ed 6. New York, Harper & Row, 1990.

38. Tortorici MR: *Fundamentals of Angiography.* St Louis, CV Mosby Co, 1982.

39. Travis E: *Primer of Medical Radiobiology,* ed 2. Chicago, Yearbook Medical Publishers, 1989.

40. Wicke L: *Atlas of Radiologic Anatomy,* ed 4. Baltimore, Urban & Schwarzenberg, 1987.